THE LEAN ADVANTAGE 3

Other books by Clarence Bass:

RIPPED
The Sensible Way to Achieve Ultimate Muscularity

RIPPED 2
The All-new Companion Volume to RIPPED

RIPPED 3
The Recipes, the Routines & the Reasons

THE LEAN ADVANTAGE
Four Years of the Ripped Question and Answer Department

THE LEAN ADVANTAGE 2
The Second Four Years

LEAN FOR LIFE
The Lifestyle Approach to Leanness

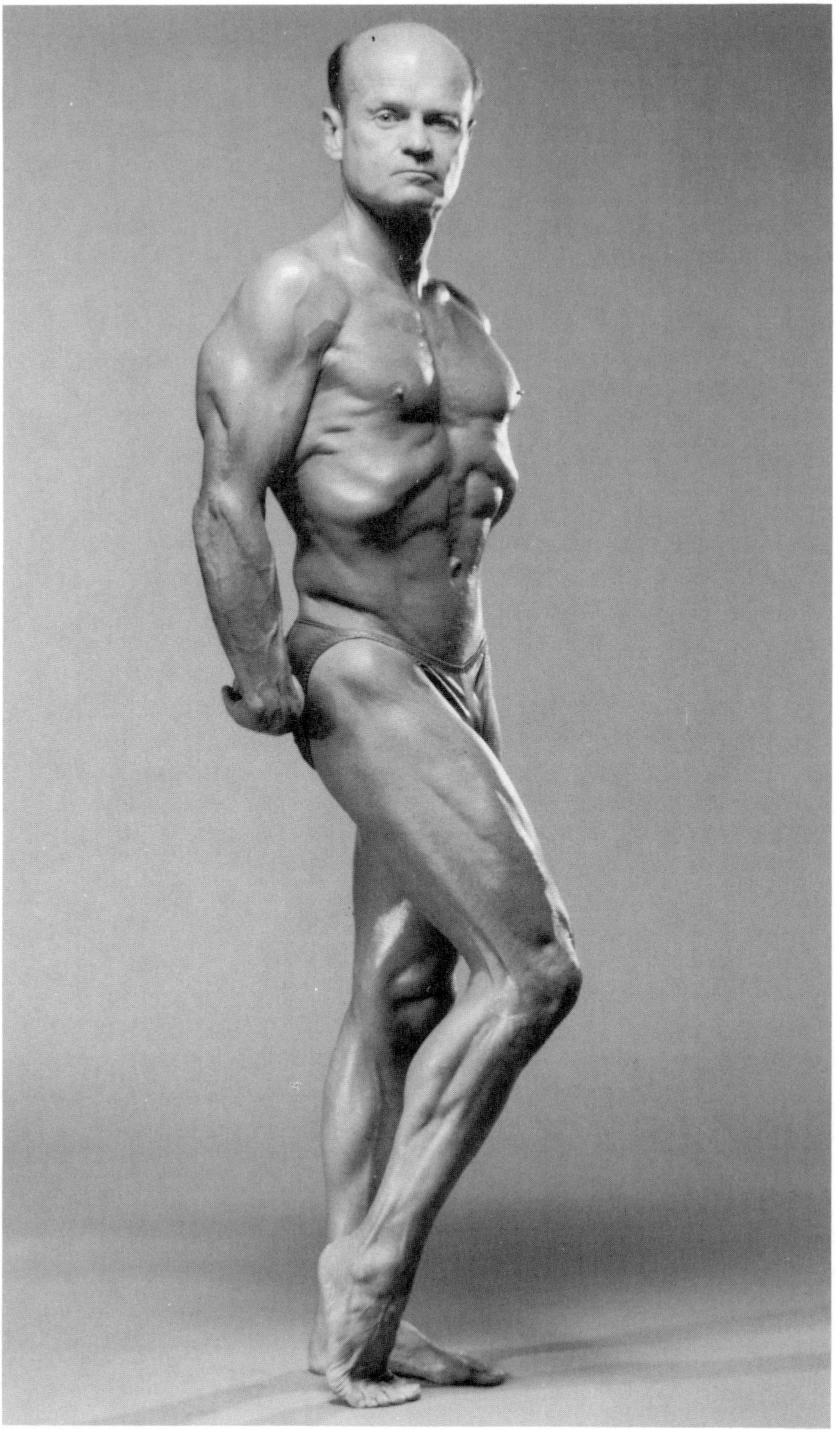

The author at 55. *Photo by Pat Berrett.*

THE LEAN ADVANTAGE 3

Four More Years

by Clarence Bass

Clarence Bass' RIPPED™ Enterprises
Albuquerque, New Mexico

ISBN 0-9609714-6-7

Published by Clarence Bass' Ripped Enterprises
528 Chama, N.E.
Albuquerque, New Mexico 87108, U.S.A.
(505) 266-5858 FAX 1-505266-9123

RIPPED is the trademark of Clarence and Carol Bass.

Library of Congress catalog card number: 84-71083

ISBN 0-9609714-6-7

Composition by Wright Graphics
Albuquerque, New Mexico

Manufactured by Thomson-Shore, Inc.
Dexter, Michigan

Photograph on front cover by John Balik
Photographs on back cover by Bill Reynolds and Pat Berrett

DEDICATION

I want to thank Joe Weider for letting me reach the millions of *Muscle & Fitness* readers around the world. Joe makes it happen. He's my friend, and I'm delighted to dedicate the entire *Lean Advantage* series to him. Thanks again Joe, for the opportunity — and your support — over the last 13 years.

WARNING

Any application of the recommendations set forth in the following pages is in the reader's discretion and sole risk.

The information in this book is intended for people in good health. If you have medical problems — of any nature — see your doctor before starting a diet and exercise program. Furthermore, even if you have no known health problems, it is advisable to consult your doctor before making any major changes in your lifestyle.

Invariably, if you are out of shape and want to start training, follow the advice of the American Medical Association: "Start *slowly* and increase the vigor and duration of the activity as your fitness improves."

ACKNOWLEDGMENTS

I'm proud of my column in *Muscle & Fitness.* I practice what I preach. I believe in what I write. And I know I've helped many people become leaner, stronger, healthier — and happier. Still, none of this happens in a vacuum. A number of people help me with the column each month, and others helped with this book. I want to acknowledge some of them here.

Thank goodness for computers; if it wasn't for our word processing program, which makes revisions easy, Carol and I would be on the verge of divorce every month. She types and corrects the column — over and over — telling me when something doesn't sound quite right. Once the column is in final form, Carol puts it on a floppy disk and sends it to computer whiz Marcella Montaner at *Muscle & Fitness.*

Executive Editor Mary Ann Mucica is the next person to receive the column. She looks it over, calls me if any further revisions are necessary, and then passes it on to Article Editors John Foster and Jo Ellen Krumm for final polishing.

Carole Wright, Wright Graphics, and Harriet "Golden Fingers" Taylor prepared *The Lean Advantage 3* for the printer. This is the sixth book we've worked on together. Harriet set the type and, as far as I'm concerned, she's the best there is; her accuracy is simply unreal. Carole helped me with the cover design and did the art work and paste-up to put the book in camera-ready form for our printer, Thomson-Shore, Inc. of Dexter, Michigan.

I thank you for all your help and support.

Finally, I want to thank the readers of *Muscle & Fitness* who write and call almost daily. They are my inspiration; their questions and comments are the catalyst each month for the Ripped Department.

TABLE OF CONTENTS

CHAPTER FIVE
WEIGHT TRAINING

CHAPTER SIX
AEROBICS

CHAPTER SEVEN
PHYSIOLOGICAL FACTORS

CHAPTER EIGHT
PSYCHOLOGICAL FACTORS

CHAPTER NINE
HEALTH FACTORS

CHAPTER TEN
THE AGE FACTOR

CHAPTER ELEVEN
THE LEAN LIFESTYLE

CHAPTER TWELVE
THE LAST WORD

INTRODUCTION

BRIDGING THE GAP

An introduction to athlete/writer Clarence Bass, the most articulate and well-read spokesman in America for an all-round fitness lifestyle, and his immensely popular Muscle & Fitness *"Ripped" column*

By David Prokop

It was the summer of 1980. I was standing outside Gold's Gym in Santa Monica, Calif. — *the* Gold's Gym, where many of the world's greatest bodybuilders, including Arnold Schwarzenegger and Lou Ferrigno, pumped iron. A long-time distance runner, I had just moved to Los Angeles to become senior editor of *Muscle & Fitness,* the leading bodybuilding publication, after several years as assistant editor of *Runner's World.* This bodybuilding environment was something totally foreign and exotic to me — and, because of that, fascinating.

Champion male bodybuilders may look tall, streamlined and aesthetic in those photos you see in the muscle magazines, but in person, whether they're wearing street clothes or workout gear, they just look *wide.* I mean, two of me could easily fit into one of them — and I'm built rather heavily for a runner. The thought that kept running through my mind that day: I've never seen so many heavily muscled guys in my life!

About the only person, other than me, on the sidewalk outside Gold's Gym that day who didn't seem to be as wide as he was tall was a bald, athletic fellow in a shirt, tie and jacket. In fact, he and I looked, at first glance, almost the same height and weight. I walked over to him and asked (more or less as a way of making conversation): "Are you a bodybuilder?"

I was somewhat embarrassed, and completely taken aback, when he replied in a calm, soft voice: "Yes, I'm the short class Past-40 Mr. America."

That's the way I first met Clarence Bass, and I guess you could say he's been my favorite bodybuilder ever since. *Him* I could relate to; those other guys with the 21-inch biceps were another matter.

As you probably guessed, Clarence didn't win that bodybuilding title on the basis of sheer muscle size. But what he lacked in size, he more than made up for in refinement — tremendous muscle definition resulting from conscientious training (weights and aerobics) and careful attention to nutrition. In bodybuilding parlance, that defined, striated look (which is a combination of having as much muscle and as little fat as possible) is called being "ripped." And Clarence was — and is — the reigning expert on attaining and maintaining that look.

Clarence's bodyfat was measured 21 times from September '79 to January '83, and averaged an amazing 3.7 percent! His lowest reading in '79 was 2.4, in '80 it was 2.7 and in '81 it was 2.4 again. By comparison, top marathon runners average approximately 6 percent bodyfat. Alberto Salazar's lowest bodyfat percentage was 5.0, Derek Clayton,s was 7.0. Frank Shorter was measured at 2.0 percent bodyfat when he won the marathon in Munich. But these guys were running upwards of 150 miles per week!

Clarence has written four narrative books explaining how to reduce bodyfat in a safe and effective way — without having to run 150 miles each week. In addition to the books, his popular and informative question-and-answer column, "Ripped," has been an ongoing feature in *Muscle & Fitness* each month since, coincidentally, the summer of 1980 — in other words, the time I first met him. The first 101 of these columns have been collected and published in two additional books, *The Lean Advantage* and *The Lean Advantage 2.* You have in hand the third collection of his columns — his seventh book in all — *The Lean Advantage 3.*

In the 13 years since I met Clarence Bass, he has become probably the most articulate and well-read spokesman in America for an all-round fitness lifestyle combining weight training, aerobics and diet. That's saying a lot, and it's important that I explain the credentials that, in my opinion, place him in that position.

Clarence first became interested in weight training when he was about 13 years old. (He's now 56.) And it enabled him to win the New Mexico High School Pentathlon championship — not the pentathlon familiar to track fans, but a five-event competition that included Chin-Ups, Push-Ups, Jump Reach, Bar Vault and 300-yard Shuttle Run. His high school athletic career also included wrestling, along with the Olympic weightlifting he did on his own.

After high school he continued with his competitive weightlifting, ultimately winning numerous regional championships and recording best lifts of 275 pounds in the Standing Press, 245 in the Snatch and 325 in the Clean and Jerk. At one time he was one of the youngest lifters in the country to lift 300 pounds in the Clean and Jerk (try to imagine what it's like lifting 300 pounds over your head!). In his late 30s he retired from competitive weightlifting and became a bodybuilder. He's been bodybuilding and writing clearly, convincingly and captivatingly about it ever since. And, somewhere in there he managed to graduate number two in his law school class and practice law — and marry and raise a family as well.

For a fellow who's been a serious weightlifter or bodybuilder all his adult life, Clarence Bass is surprisingly knowledgeable about aerobics. He has been a *Runner's World* subscriber for over 20 years. And for a decade after he first read Dr. Kenneth Cooper's landmark book *Aerobics* in the late '60s and became sold on the benefits of aerobic exercise, Clarence ran fairly regularly, achieving a personal goal of running under six minutes for the mile ("I did 5:50").

"When I first started doing aerobic exercise, what I did, of course, was running," Clarence says. "I didn't know of any other kind of aerobic exercise frankly at that point. And I ran for about 10 years — from about '68 to '78. Then I finally gravitated into riding a bike, and as I got involved in learning more about total body aerobics, I got into the Air-Dyne, which is the stationary bike I have here which has the push-pull arm action. And I've gotten even more involved in that whole body concept lately with the rower. I also have a Versa-Climber and a Nordic Track. And, of course, I've been involved in the HeavyHands concept (where you do endurance exercise with light hand weights in your hands). But I definitely started with the running."

Clarence's column and books are filled with references to running and people who excel at it or write about it. "I've always been interested in seeing how the runners do things," Clarence says, "and in many cases I've transported what the runners do over to the bodybuilding field and it has worked well. One thing that sticks out in my mind is the hard-day/easy-day training approach, which I think is something that former Oregon track coach Bill Bowerman first started. In the past, bodybuilders have been inclined to go to the gym and train all out every time. From the runners, I borrowed the idea that every time you really have a hard training session, you need to follow it with one or maybe two easier sessions in order to get maximum benefit, and that concept has worked successfully.

"As I got further along in my aerobic training, I became interested in reading about runners and other aerobic athletes using cross-training, say, at times when they were injured or when they just wanted to add variety to their training. Then I read the HeavyHands book by Dr. Leonard Schwartz, where he talks about whole body aerobic exercise, training your upper body as well as your lower body. And I've been able to adapt that to the bodybuilding field and understand more about the physiology of exercise. One thing I learned is that the changes that take place in your muscles as a result of exercise take place only in the muscles you're using. So by training your upper body aerobically (as in cross-country skiing or on the Air-Dyne stationary bike, where you work the arms as well as the legs), you have the changes take place there as well as in the legs, which is what is used exclusively in most aerobic exercise.

"I think I've always been interested in reading everything (on fitness, training and nutrition) that I can get my hands on," says Clarence. "But when I started doing the 'Ripped' column in *Muscle & Fitness,* that was an additional prod because I now had to come up with something new each month. That was easy at first, but as it went on, it started becoming harder, so I had to search out new things. Of course, that made me look at the running magazines much more carefully, and I got a lot of ideas that I ended up using in the column. And I'm always looking for new diet books or new training books. Plus, I'm a long time subscriber to *The Physician and Sportsmedicine,* and multiple newsletters and magazines in the sports, health and fitness fields.

"I constantly have my antennae out to find new things that I can bring back to my field. I try to be careful in my writing not to get out of my area of expertise. I think of my area of expertise as being how to get lean and stay that way. So I try to pick and choose things that I can bring to that field, and then stir it up or integrate it into my own experience and hopefully come up with something that is interesting and informative to the readers.

"And as the column has gone along, I've broadened my approach to bring in more health aspects — more of a total fitness-health approach."

You'll notice that when Clarence talks about his area of expertise, he makes no mention of his extensive knowledge about weight training, bodybuilding or aerobic exercise. That's because in his view, being an expert on getting lean and staying that way *encompasses* knowledge about weight training and aerobics. It all goes together — nutrition, weight training and aerobics.

Clarence's father was a doctor, and so was his grandfather and great-grandfather. So you could say Clarence comes by his interest in health and fitness naturally. Maybe that also helps explain why he's become such a dedicated researcher in his field, a thinking man's writer whose ever broadening perspective has made his work relevant to anyone interested in health, fitness and weight loss — or weight maintenance.

He once explained to me in a letter: "I like to think that I write for a thinking audience. I always want to know why, so in my writing I try to explain the 'why' in the same way I'd like to have someone explain it to me. I want it to make so much sense, be so clear and persuasive, that it becomes obvious that it's the right approach."

As we all noticed, times have changed. Back in the '50s, '60s and even into the '70s, runners ran, swimmers swam, cyclists cycled and bodybuilders pumped iron. There wasn't much overlap of these activities. But with the flowering of our fitness consciousness in the last decade or so, there's been an interesting cross-pollination of information from one activity or sport to another. A new consciousness is emerging. More bodybuilders are now running and doing other aerobic activities. And, in turn, we're seeing more runners — and athletes in all sports — weight training than ever before. The fitness trend of the '90s is clearly to use the best of both worlds. Thanks to people like Clarence Bass, we're finally bridging the gap.

CHAPTER ONE

BODYFAT TESTS

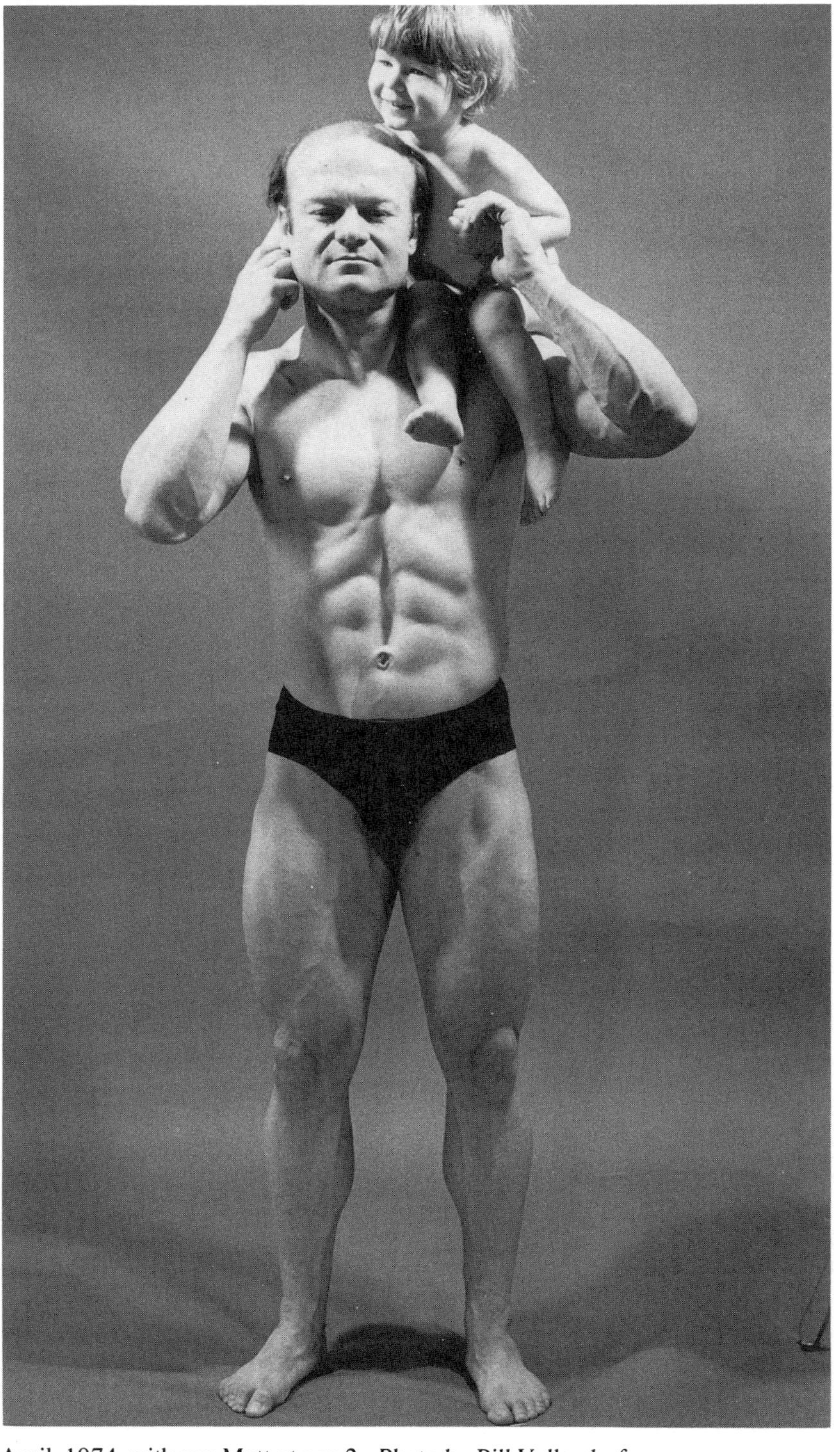

April, 1974, with son Matt at age 2. *Photo by Bill Vollendorf.*

BODYFAT TESTS 1

WHAT'S YOUR BODYFAT?

Find out by using the hydrostatic, skinfold, impedance, ultrasound or infrared methods

Bodyfat testing has come out of the lab and into the mainstream of the fitness lifestyle. Bodyfat is a hot topic in the gym these days. More people than ever before know their bodyfat percentage — or at least that it's important. Bodyweight is out. What counts is bodyfat level, body composition, how much of your weight is muscle and how much is fat. Still, some little-understood problems remain that bodybuilders and fitness enthusiasts need to know about. Sometimes bodyfat tests are not all they're cracked up to be. On the other hand, some exciting — and positive — new developments have come on the scene.

Properly used and understood, body composition tests can be a great help in training. Your bathroom scale doesn't tell you whether the weight you lost or gained is fat or muscle. What's more, desirable changes can take place in your body even if your weight stays the same. Your scale may indicate nothing is happening when, in fact, you're replacing fat with muscle. In these circumstances, body composition tests come to your aid; they quantify your progress.

Training Boon

Body composition tests help guide your training. At the outset, they tell you how much of your bodyweight is lean and how much is fat. Your mirror says whether you're too fat, and a body composition test gives you the details. It tells you how many pounds of fat you need to lose. After you embark on a diet and exercise program, further tests give you the feedback needed to zero in on your goal.

Since 1977, when I was first tested at Lovelace Medical Center in Albuquerque, body composition tests have been a critical part of my training regimen. The tests tell me when I'm doing things right and, equally important, when I'm doing things wrong. I always keep an eye on the scale, but I never forget that bodyweight changes are made up of lean tissue and fat tissue. Rarely are gains all muscle or losses all fat. If you want the whole story on the results of your training, body composition tests are essential.

There's a slight catch, however. All methods used to measure bodyfat are indirect. (Direct measurement would require that you be dissected and subjected to compositional analysis.) All body composition tests are estimates. They are based on assumptions that can vary from one testing method to the next and even within a single method. This being the case, if you're not careful you can end up comparing apples and oranges. This is true even with underwater (hydrostatic) weighing, the most reliable and generally accepted method for determining body composition. It's the gold standard by which other techniques are judged.

Shocking Discrepancies

To demonstrate the problem, I had doctoral candidate Kay Steffens weigh me underwater at the University of New Mexico Human Performance Laboratory and estimate my bodyfat using different procedures and assumptions. Even Kay, who has 11 years experience in body composition testing and has weighed me at regular intervals since 1984, found the discrepancies shocking.

Using one technique, the most accurate procedure according to Steffens and the UNM lab, my bodyfat was estimated to be 3.9%. Several other commonly used techniques, however, placed my bodyfat level as high as 10.7%. That's a huge variation. A fat level of 10.7% would mean I was carrying 10 pounds more fat (and 10 pounds less muscle) than indicated by the best and most accurate procedure. What caused this startling difference?

Underwater Weighing

Underwater weighing is based on the fact that fat is not as dense as lean body mass and tends to float while the latter, with its bone and muscle, is denser and tends to sink. Your bodyweight out of water is compared to your weight completely submerged. As you become leaner and more muscular, you become denser and heavier in relation to the water your body displaces. While a fat person floats like a beachball, a lean person sinks like a cannonball.

The amount of air in the lungs, of course, has an effect on your underwater weight. It makes you comparatively buoyant. Some air remains in the lungs even after you blow out all you can. Hydrostatic weighing, therefore, attempts to take into account the air in the lungs after a maximum expiration. There are two ways to do this. Residual lung volume can be measured by an open circuit nitrogen washout technique or by a closed-circuit oxygen or helium dilution method.

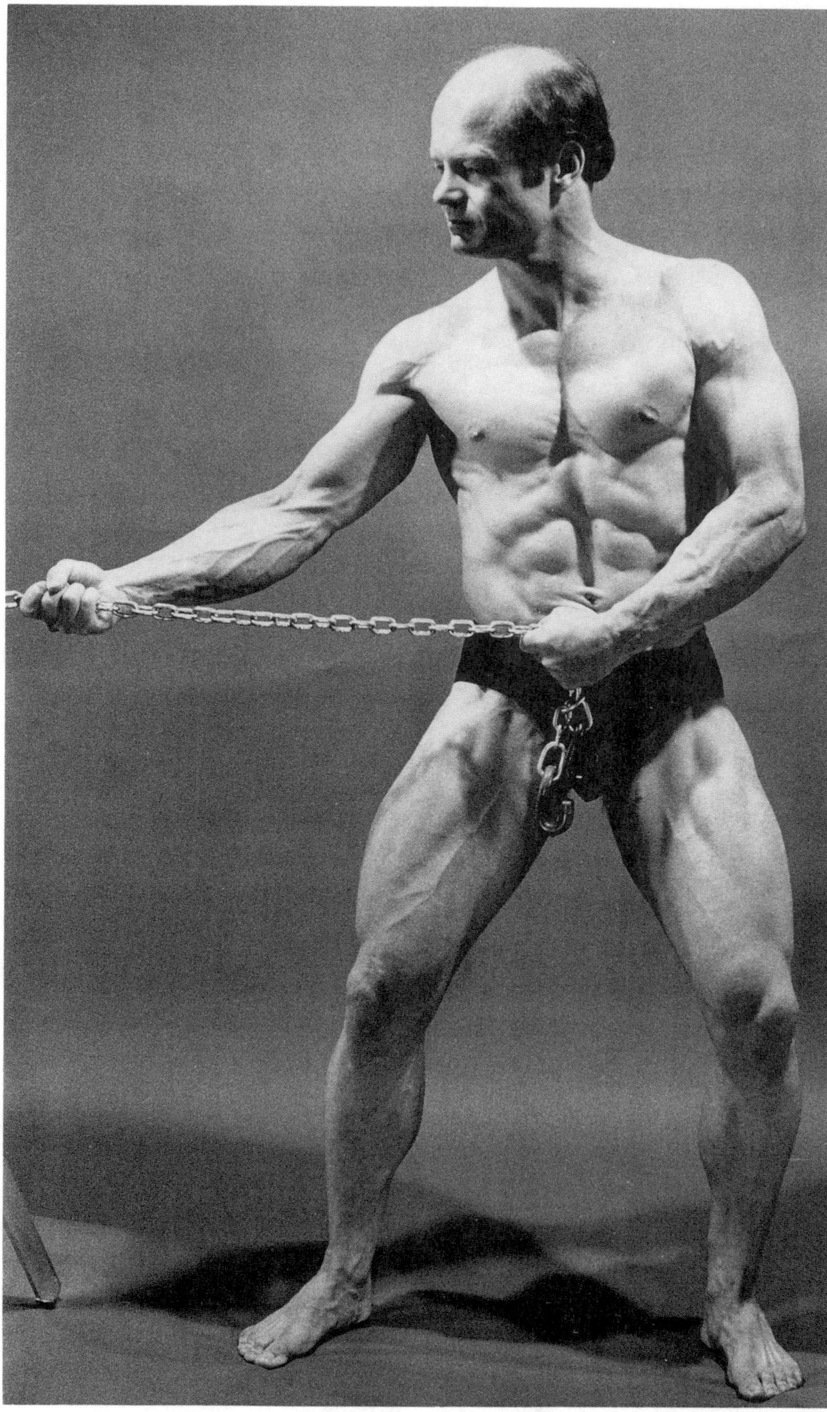

This photo is one of my first attempts at physique photography. It was taken by my next door neighbor, *Bill Vollendorf*, in 1974.

More often, however, it is estimated. This is understandable, because actually measuring residual lung volume can add as much as $100 to the cost of hydrostatic weighing.

Still, this is unfortunate, because Professors William D. McArdle, Frank I. Katch and Victor L. Katch tell us in their textbook *Exercise Physiology* (Lea & Febiger, 1986) that residual lung volume is large and variable among subjects. As confirmed by Drs. Pollock, Wilmore and Fox in *Exercise in Health and Disease* (W.B. Saunders Co., 1984), errors in residual volume can make a dramatic difference in the results. That difference, the difference between estimating and measuring the air in the lungs, explains part of the disparate results of my recent weighing.

Measuring Lung Volume

Frankly, I hadn't realized how much difference it could make to estimate the air in the lungs. When Lovelace Medical Center determined my body composition the first time, in 1977, they measured my actual residual lung volume. In 1984, when I went to the University of New Mexico for testing, my residual volume was again measured. My tests, in the past, have always been based on measured residual volume.

"For screening purposes or when measuring large groups, the estimate of [residual volume] would be an acceptable technique," says Dr. Pollock and his colleagues. They go on to state, however, that "[residual volume] is quite variable in any given age, height, or vital capacity and may result in errors of up to five percent bodyfat." For individual analysis and counseling, they recommend that residual volume be measured, not estimated.

In my case, Steffens found that predicting residual lung volume, according to the recommended formula developed by Goldman and Becklake, increased my estimated fat weight to 9.5 pounds from 6 pounds, an increase of almost 60%! And that's only part of the discrepancy that showed up in my weighings.

The additional difference also had to do with air in the lungs. A commonly used technique is to have the subject make a forced maximal exhalation as the head is lowered under the surface. This takes practice. It's hard — and a little scary — to purge all the air from one's lungs underwater, and then sit still while the weight is recorded. Recognizing this problem, Dr. Ulrich C. Luft and T.P.K. Lim of the Lovelace Medical Center developed a modified procedure. Details can be found in "Techniques for Measuring Body Composition," National Academy of Science, National Research Council, Washington, D.C., 1961, page 107. In simplified terms, you fill your lungs with air, expire a *measured amount,* then duck your head under the surface and remain motionless while your weight is recorded. The difference is that you're not required to blow all your air out. They let you keep some air in your lungs, and then measure it using a spirometer.

The University of New Mexico Human Performance Laboratory adopted this method. Kay Steffens has always used the modified procedure for my weighings. It's much easier on the subject, believe me, and Kay says the results are more consistent and reliable. She believes it's difficult for most people to blow out all their air while bent over underwater. Plus, even a small amount of unaccounted-for air can play havoc with the test.

My results confirm this. When I attempted to blow all the air out of my lungs, my bodyfat percentage came out 8.3%, or 4.4% more than when the modified procedure was used. That's using my actual measured residual volume. When my predicted residual volume was used, and in addition I attempted to empty my lungs underwater, my bodyfat level came out 10.7%. Altogether, unanticipated air added 6.8% (10.7% minus 3.9%) to my estimated fat level. So you see, different weighing techniques can make a huge difference.

The important point, however, is not that a particular method is best, but the fact that different measuring techniques can alter the test results dramatically. When you have your body composition tested, be sure the same technique is used every time. That way you'll be comparing apples and apples, not apples and oranges. In my case, I've always been tested the same way. This allows me to accurately follow the changes in my body composition. If I allowed the measuring technique to change from one weighing to the next, the results would be meaningless.

To give you an idea of the cost of underwater weighing, the UNM Human Performance Laboratory charges $35. The Cooper Clinic in Dallas, as part of a complete medical and fitness evaluation, charges $28 for underwater weighing. Profit organizations like Lovelace Medical Center usually charge more, up to $100.

As I've already indicated, having residual lung volume measured, rather than estimated, can add another $100 to the cost of hydrostatic weighing. Nevertheless, I believe the added accuracy makes the extra expense worthwhile. After all, it's basically a one-time expense. Your residual volume is good for several years; it can be used over and over in subsequent weighings.

The drawback of underwater weighing is that it requires expensive equipment, a trained administrator and considerable cooperation by the subject. Still, it's the most accurate method, with a 3-4% margin of error for most people.

Skinfold Measurement

Skinfold thickness is one of the simplest ways to measure body composition. It doesn't require costly equipment or a laboratory setting. It uses relatively inexpensive calipers to estimate fatness based on the thickness of the fat under the skin. For most people, the skinfold technique is accurate to plus or minus 5% when measurements are taken properly in several sites (usually four different sites). If you're very fat or very lean, however, the margin of error can be higher. I'll use myself again to show how the results can vary.

As I've explained, all body composition tests are based on assumptions. This, of course, includes skinfolds. Older people, like me, are assumed to have less muscle and more internal fat than younger people. It should come as no surprise, therefore, that the Cooper Clinic estimated my bodyfat at 7.5% using skinfold calibration and my age, 51. Using the assumptions for a 35-year-old, however, I was 5.5% by skinfold. Finally, considered as a 20-year-old, I was 3.7%. The last figure, you'll recall, is about where the UNM lab put my bodyfat based on underwater weighing. In short, the age-based assumptions can skew the results for some people, including many bodybuilders who don't fit the norms.

Again, the important thing is to use the same assumptions all the time. Pick the criterion that fits your case best, and stick with that measure in all future tests. Remember, apples and apples.

The University of New Mexico charges the general public $10 for skinfold measurement. Profit organizations typically charge more.

That brings us to the new high-tech methods: electrical impedance, ultrasound and infrared.

Electrical Impedance

The electrical impedance technique for measuring bodyfat was first written up in *Muscle & Fitness* several years ago, and I've followed it with great interest. Body composition analyzers utilizing this method are found in many gyms, health food stores, medical clinics and elsewhere. Many facilities use the device as a traffic builder; they'll measure your bodyfat for a small charge, about the same as skinfold measurements, or even for free. What are the pros and cons of this technique?

The electrical impedance method is based on the principle that the electrical conductivity of lean tissue is far greater than that of fat. Fat offers more resistance than lean tissue to an electrical current passed through the body.

According to a number of research studies I've read, the impedance technique is promising. The advantage is not that it's more accurate than other methods. As I've said, underwater weighing is the most accurate technique. All other methods are judged on the basis of their correlation to hydrostatic weighing. But as we already know, hydrostatic weighing is a complicated procedure.

That's where electrical impedance has an advantage. It's fast and convenient. It requires no special skill on the part of the operator or the subject and takes only a few minutes. The procedure is simple: Electrodes are placed on the wrist and ankle and a weak electrical charge is passed through the body. There are some problems, however.

Because water is a main component of lean tissue, this method relies heavily on the fact that water is an excellent conductor of electricity. According to *The Physician and Sportsmedicine,* this may be the Achilles' heel of the impedance technique. Apparently impedance testing does not — and may be unable to — allow for the natural variation in body water among individuals.

Timothy G. Lohman, Ph.D., professor in the department of exercise and sportsmedicine at the University of Arizona, Tucson, said: "It's apparent that exercise, dehydration, and eating and drinking affect impedance. Readings are totally off when the body's water compartments are high or low."

Larry R. Gettman, Ph.D., director of the Vita Health & Fitness Center in Plano, Texas, reported: "I've tried impedance testing with [the Dallas Cowboys] and all the lean players had high fat readings, while all the fat players had low readings. . . . Extremes are way off. . . . I measured one fellow at 40% bodyfat using impedance, and he measured only 15% with skinfold calipers."

Arno L. Jensen, MD, a radiologist and preventive medicine specialist at the Cooper Clinic, agrees with this assessment. Still, Jensen believes that electrical impedance has value for the broad range of people who are neither extremely lean or fat. He has one of the devices in his office and uses it routinely, along with underwater weighing and skinfolds.

When I was at the Cooper Clinic for my second evaluation last September, Jensen measured my bodyfat using electrical impedance. The results seemed to confirm the erratic results for people at the extremes and when water balance is disturbed. My initial reading was 2.5%, but Jensen didn't feel that this was accurate, because I had just completed the treadmill test and was somewhat dehydrated. When he checked me again after I had eaten, the result was 8.5%. That's probably high.

So the results of the electrical impedance method can be somewhat variable. Nevertheless, this method is quite acceptable for most people. In fact, a study published in the *American Journal of Clinical Nutrition* (1988; 47: 7-14) involving 1,567 adults aged 17-62 and with 3-56% bodyfat came to this conclusion: Bioelectrical impedance analysis "is a rapid, non-invasive, and convenient method for nutritional assessment of healthy individuals and groups."

The only caution I would add is the same as for other techniques: For meaningful assessment of body composition changes using electrical impedance you must be tested using the same assumptions and under the same circumstances.

Ultrasound

I have no personal experience with the ultrasound method of body composition analysis. Nevertheless, I believe it has merit.

The idea behind this technique is the same as skinfold thickness. The difference is that the fatfolds are measured not by calipers, but by passing sound waves through adipose tissue until the muscle is reached. Ultrasound measurements are taken at four or five sites, just like regular fatfold assessment.

The weakness of the technique is the same as calipers: The measurements are only as good as the assumptions used. On the other hand, the measurement of fatfolds by sound waves is more accurate than calipers, especially in the obese individual.

Like calipers and impedance, this technique has an advantage over hydrostatic weighing in several respects: It's less difficult, less expensive, requires less equipment and much less of the subject.

It may also have an advantage over impedance, because fat tissue thickness doesn't change as the result of exercise or eating; it's unaffected by changes in body water level. Plus, it's faster than calipers, because the calculations are made by computer.

The bottom line is that ultrasound accurately measures what it says it measures — subcutaneous fat. That means it's as good as skinfolds for assessing bodyfat level, and probably somewhat better, because the measurement is more precise.

Infrared

Finally, the infrared technique may be the most exciting of all. Not because it's more accurate — it's not — but because it's the simplest of the bunch. You can even test yourself. All you do is punch in your personal data (sex, current weight, body frame, height and exercise level), and then apply the light wand between the shoulder and elbow on the biceps of your dominant arm. That's it, one reading, and presto, out comes your bodyfat percentage.

This method uses a technology developed by the U.S. Department of Agriculture to measure the fat content of meat. A light beam enters the body and the presence of fat changes the spectrum of the light beam. Bodyfat percentage is estimated by measuring the spectrum shift.

Like skinfolds and ultrasound, infrared measurements were first taken at several locations, but then it was discovered that a reading taken from the biceps alone was a good predictor of overall bodyfat. In fact, several research studies indicate that this single site measurement predicts bodyfat level about as well as traditional skinfold measurements. A study in Sweden determined that the correlation between the two techniques was almost 90%.

Conclusion

My bodyfat percentage as measured by the infrared technique is 1-2% higher than by underwater weighing as performed at the UNM lab. I could adjust the readout on the infrared unit to coincide with my bodyfat as measured hydrostatically, but I have decided against it. My reason is what this article is about. It's the bottom line on bodyfat tests.

While I was at the Cooper Clinic, Jensen introduced me to John J. Duncan, their expert on body composition analysis. It took Duncan only a few sentences to put bodyfat tests in proper perspective. Body composition tests are not exact, he says. "The whole field is based on the study of about 40 cadavers, all white men, no women and no blacks." It's all very tenuous, but he says that's okay.

Duncan, you see, doesn't require absolute accuracy. It doesn't make a whole lot of difference to him whether a patient's bodyfat is precisely 15% or 20%. His concern is measuring the change that takes place as a result of intervention. In other words, he wants to be able to assess whether diet and exercise prescriptions are having the desired effect. Properly administered, he believes body composition tests do that pretty well.

Bodyfat tests work for Duncan. And they'll work for you, too, as long as you remember that it's not absolute accuracy that's important in bodyfat testing; it's the accurate assessment of change. In the final analysis, all the methods we've discussed — hydrostatic, skinfold, impedance, ultrasound and infrared — will perform that function satisfactorily.

Jensen sums it up this way: "The way to use percent bodyfat is to pick one of the methods and use it consistently, under the same circumstances, to monitor various training or diet regimens."

GOVERNMENT COP-OUT

New age-based weight tables misguided

There they go again. First, the federal government procrastinated for more than 20 years before endorsing the 1968 American Heart Association recommendation that we get no more than 30% of our calories from fat. Now they're telling us that middle-aged spread is okay.

The U.S. Department of Agriculture and Health and Human Services have issued new "health-based weight criteria" suggesting that a 10-or 15-pound gain after age 34 is acceptable. The new government weight tables have one set of recommendations for ages 19-34, and a second and heavier range for 35 and over. For example, the government says a 5′9″ man should weigh between 129 and 169 pounds until age 34, but after that a range of 142 to 183 is satisfactory.

Granted, that's what usually happens. On average, Americans accumulate an extra pound or two a year between the ages of 20 and 50. The question, however, is whether it's healthy to gain weight with age. The new government-approved weight ranges suggest that it is. In my opinion, that's a cop-out.

Researchers such as Dr. Dean Ornish have shown that we would be leaner and healthier, and probably live longer, if we consumed only 20% — or better still 10% — of our calories in fat. Nevertheless, the government recommends 30%. Why? Because they know that the typical American diet is 40-50% fat, and they don't think people will be willing to cut fat intake as much as they really should. So they settle for 30%.

Weight Tables

The same type of thinking seems to be at work in the new age-based weight tables. Government researchers know full well that it's best not to gain weight with age. Nevertheless, they think that's too much to ask, that people are unlikely to change their lifestyle to that extent. So they compromise again and urge that we restrict after-35 weight gain to about 10%. The message from the government seems to be: "Mediocre is good enough."

I don't buy it. Let me tell you why.

First, for sedentary people weight gained after 25 is almost always fat. In fact, even those who weigh the same at 40 as they did at 20 are usually fatter. That's because people who don't exercise lose muscle as they age and replace it with fat. It goes without saying, of course, that most people who gain weight after 35, as permitted by the new government tables, actually gain more fat than weight.

Covert Bailey, in his marvelous little book *Fit Or Fat?* (Houghton Mifflin, 1977), says that a person's "correct weight" changes as lean mass changes. Bailey explains that the amount of lean body mass one has largely determines how much one can eat without gaining weight. That's because it's the lean tissue, muscle, that burns the calories we eat. Fat, for all practical purposes, doesn't need calories. That means that if two people eat the same number of calories, the one who has the least amount of muscle will gain the most weight.

It stands to reason, then, that the new government tables are going in the wrong direction. Most people lose muscles as they age and, therefore, should lose weight as well. Otherwise, they'll simply get fatter as each year goes by. That, of course, is what usually happens, and it's not good.

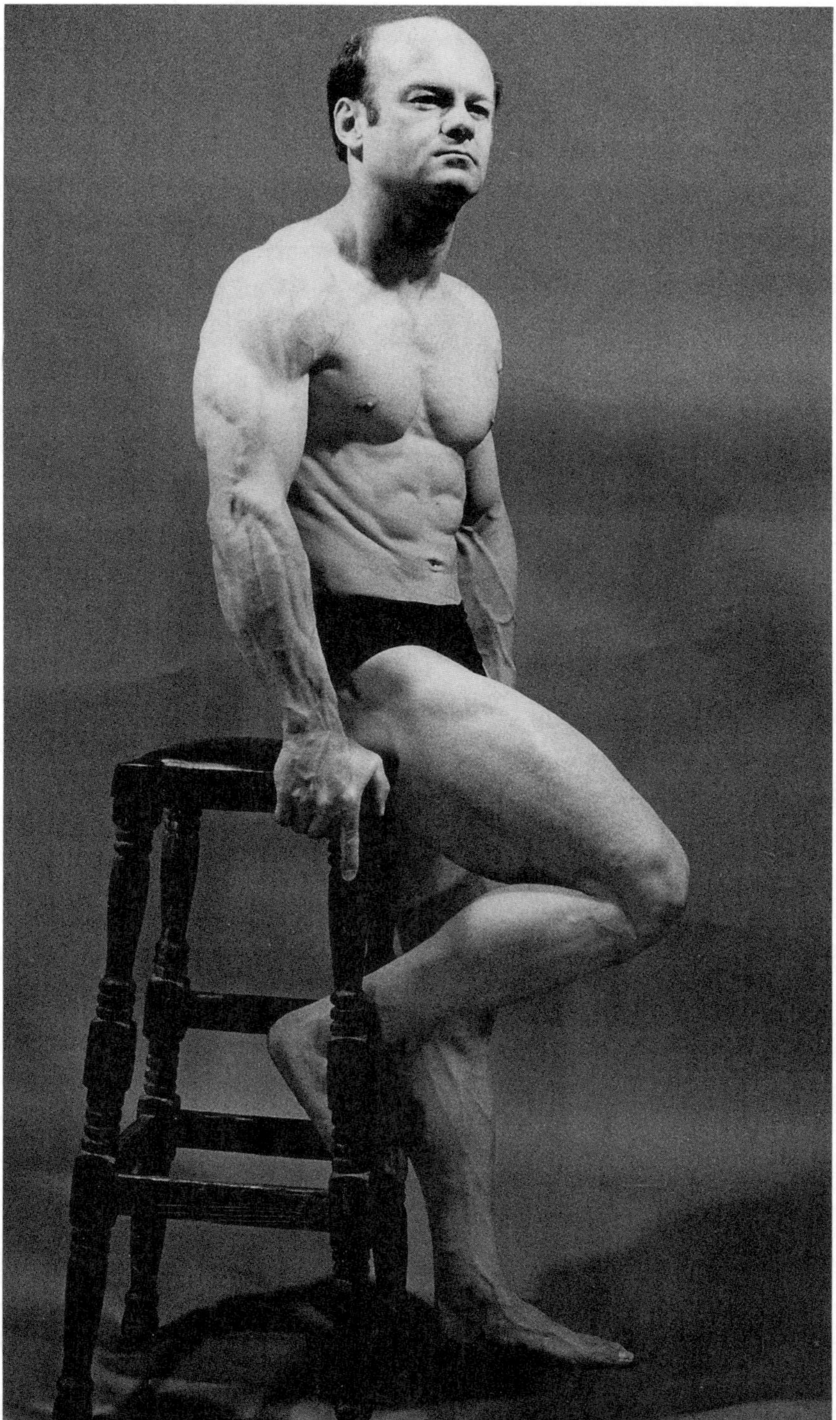

Another photo by *Bill Vollendorf*, shortly after my interest turned to bodybuilding.

Excess Fat

Excess fat is a problem at any age, but it's worse as you get older. This was borne out by the review of 25 studies on obesity conducted by Dr. JoAnn Manson and her associates at the Harvard School of Public Health reported in the Jan. 16, 1987 *Journal of the American Medical Association.* According to Manson, the studies show that the risk of death increases with weight gain. Significantly, the risk grows with age. Specifically, for people aged 30-49 the risk of death increased by 1% for each pound of excess weight, but for those in the 50-62 age range each pound increased the death rate by 2%!

It seems pretty clear then, doesn't it, that the government should be encouraging us to lose weight as we get older.

Lawrence E. Lamb, MD, a fellow *M&F* columnist and a medical consultant to the President's Council on Physical Fitness and Sports, seems to agree with me. In *The Weighting Game* (Lyle Stuart, 1988) Lamb offers this suggestion for determining how fat you are: "You can strip and look at yourself in the mirror... along with remembering what you weighed when you were 25 years old."

Before the government doctors put out the next revision of the weight tables, I wish they would read "Why Your Patients Shouldn't Take Aging Sitting Down" in the November, 1990 issue of *The Physician & Sportsmedicine.* That article argues that doctors should urge their patients to resist the natural tendency to become less active with age. Importantly, the sports-and-fitness-minded medical journal warns that people need to be especially vigilant between the ages of 30-40 — the very time when the new government tables say it's all right to let the pounds pile on. "It's the old concept of use it or lose it," explained Frederick T. Sherman, MD, an internist and geriatrician in Huntington, New York.

"Age Vigorously"

Sherman maintains that aging gracefully is for the birds. "Aging gracefully has traditionally meant sitting back in your chair and reading a book...," he says. "We want to get people out of that mindset and into a more active one. What we want to tell them is to age *vigorously.*"

Maintaining your muscle mass and your weight as you age is not all that difficult. Attention, government experts, here's the formula:

1) Eat a low-fat, high-fiber, balanced diet.
2) Do aerobic exercise to burn fat.
3) Lift weights to build and maintain muscle.

SETTING THE BODYWEIGHT STANDARD

Why it isn't normal to be average

Q: *I've been experimenting with various training and diet cycles in an effort to get my weight under control.*

My most recent approach involved three week-long diet cycles. I started each cycle by fasting completely for 24 hours, consuming nothing but water. I thought this would force my body to burn fat. My first meal coming off the fast was mostly fat. Again, I thought this would condition my body to utilize fat. For the rest of the week I ate mainly carbs, but only enough to satisfy my hunger. I lost an average of 4 pounds a week on this regimen, 12 pounds total.

Before that I lost 15 pounds with endurance workouts and a low-fat diet, but I gained 5 pounds back.

Do you think I'm on the right track with my one-week cycles?

A: No. You've succeeded in losing weight fast, but that may be your downfall in the long run. The fact that you gained weight between the two periods of dieting is a bad sign. Unfortunately, the majority of people who lose weight fast regain what they lose, and often more. They try again and again, only to find that in the long run they end up getting fatter. Yo-yo dieting is not only frustrating, recent evidence suggests that it's unhealthy.

Let me tell you about the research and some other developments — both good and bad — in the area of weight control. We seem to be getting a little better handle on the process all the time. Significantly, we're developing a new realism that should help people like you achieve and maintain desirable body weight.

Yo-Yo Dieting Dangers

A study that appeared this past summer in *The New England Journal of Medicine* suggests that repeated cycles of weight loss and gain may actually be life-threatening. In a study of 3,130 men and women, ages 30-62, Yale University psychologist Kelly Brownell found that those whose weight went up and down most over a 14-year period had a 70% higher risk of dying from heart disease than those whose weight remained relatively stable — even if they were overweight. One explanation for this is that weight may be lost mostly from the lower part of the body but gained back in the upper part. This is bad because fat from the belly is more easily mobilized and sent into the blood stream, where it can clog vital blood vessels.

Brownell believes yo-yo dieting may be most dangerous, not for people who are vastly overweight, but for people who are continuously battling those last 5 or 10 excess pounds. "These people are fighting their own biology," he says.

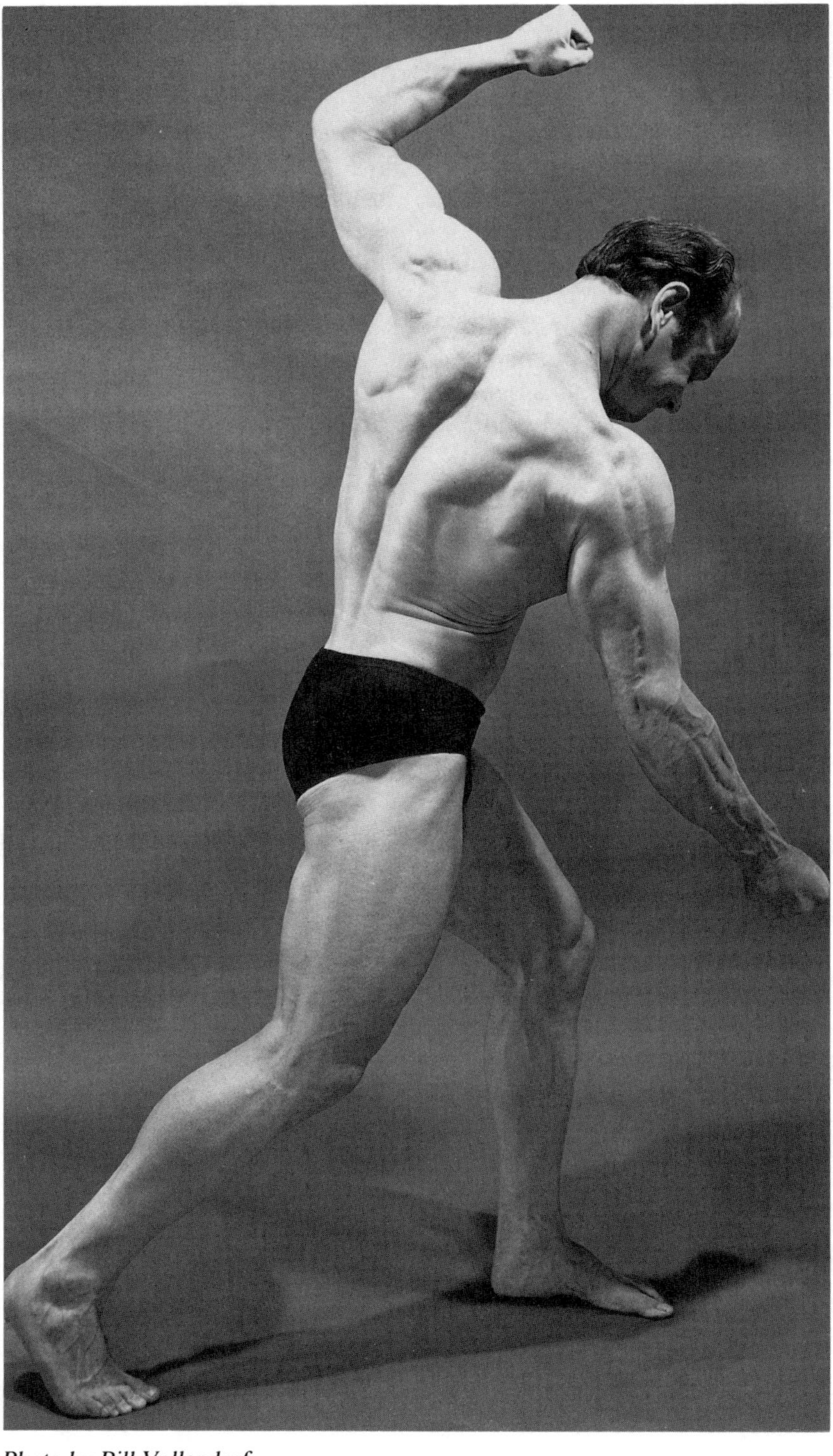

Photo by Bill Vollendorf.

It seems that each time a person sheds pounds and then puts them back on, he or she ends up with more bodyfat and less lean muscle. That's especially true for people who are already relatively lean. (Bodybuilders who bulk up between contests, take note.) Their efforts to lose weight over and over cause their body to give up muscle and lay down more fat. This is not only unhealthy, but makes it more difficult to maintain the loss, because less muscle means a slower metabolism.

In the last decade, evidence has come to light that suggests that some people are predisposed to weigh more than others. They're just not cut out to be as lean as they might like. For instance, University of Pennsylvania obesity researcher Albert Stunkard, M.D., has found that identical twins raised in different environments by different sets of parents are both likely to end up overweight (or underweight). This highlights the powerful role played by genetics. Some people are simply more prone than others to be overweight.

Unisex Weight Tables

In keeping with the trend to allow more latitude in how much we should weigh, the federal government has published new tables for "healthy" weights. Unfortunately, as so often happens, the government may have overreacted.

The new standards, published November 1990 by the Departments of Agriculture and Health & Human Services, allow for a range of 30 pounds or more at each height and up to a 16-pound gain after age 35. All people are divided into two age groups, 19-34 and 35 or older, and given a recommended weight according to height. Believe it or not, no distinction is made for males and females.

The new ideal weights are higher than those previously recommended and, as indicated, allow for increased weight in the older age group. Dr. William P. Castelli, director of the long-term Framingham Heart Study, has criticized the new recommendations.

"I don't think it's a smart idea to allow Americans to weigh 10% more. If anything they should weigh 10% less. The table says that if you are 5-foot-9, you can weigh up to 183 pounds. Well, unless you have the biggest bones on earth, you're overweight." (Some male bodybuilders, of course, weigh that much or more in lean condition.)

Lawrence E. Lamb, M.D., a fellow *M&F* columnist, agreed with Castelli. "The new unisex weight tables are a step backward," he wrote in *The Health Letter*. The Framingham Heart Study, Lamb explained, showed that every excess pound counts. In men 30-49, each pound of excess weight increased the death rate by 1%. For those aged 50-62, each pound increases the death rate by 2%.

Activity Level — Not Age

Plus, according to weight control experts William D. McArdle, Frank I. Katch and Victor L. Katch, in the third edition of *Exercise Physiology* (Lea & Febiger, 1991): "There is probably no biologic reason for men and women to get fatter as they grow older." Increases in bodyfat, according to these authors, are more a function of activity level than age.

It's true, people tend to get fatter as they grow older. It doesn't have to be that way according to the authors, who caution that *average* should not be accepted as *normal.* They believe, and I agree, that there should be only one criterion for what is considered "too fat," and that standard should apply to young and old alike.

On another matter, however, the new government guidelines are right on target. They recommend that people reduce weight at a safe rate of one-half to 1 pound per week. That's down from their previous recommendation of 1-2 pounds per week. In the weight loss game, my experience is that slow and steady wins the race.

The only realistic way to reach your ideal weight and stay there is to adopt a lifestyle that includes sensible — and comfortable — eating habits and regular exercise (aerobics and weight training). That's the formula I recommend.

CHAPTER TWO

DIET: THE BIG PICTURE

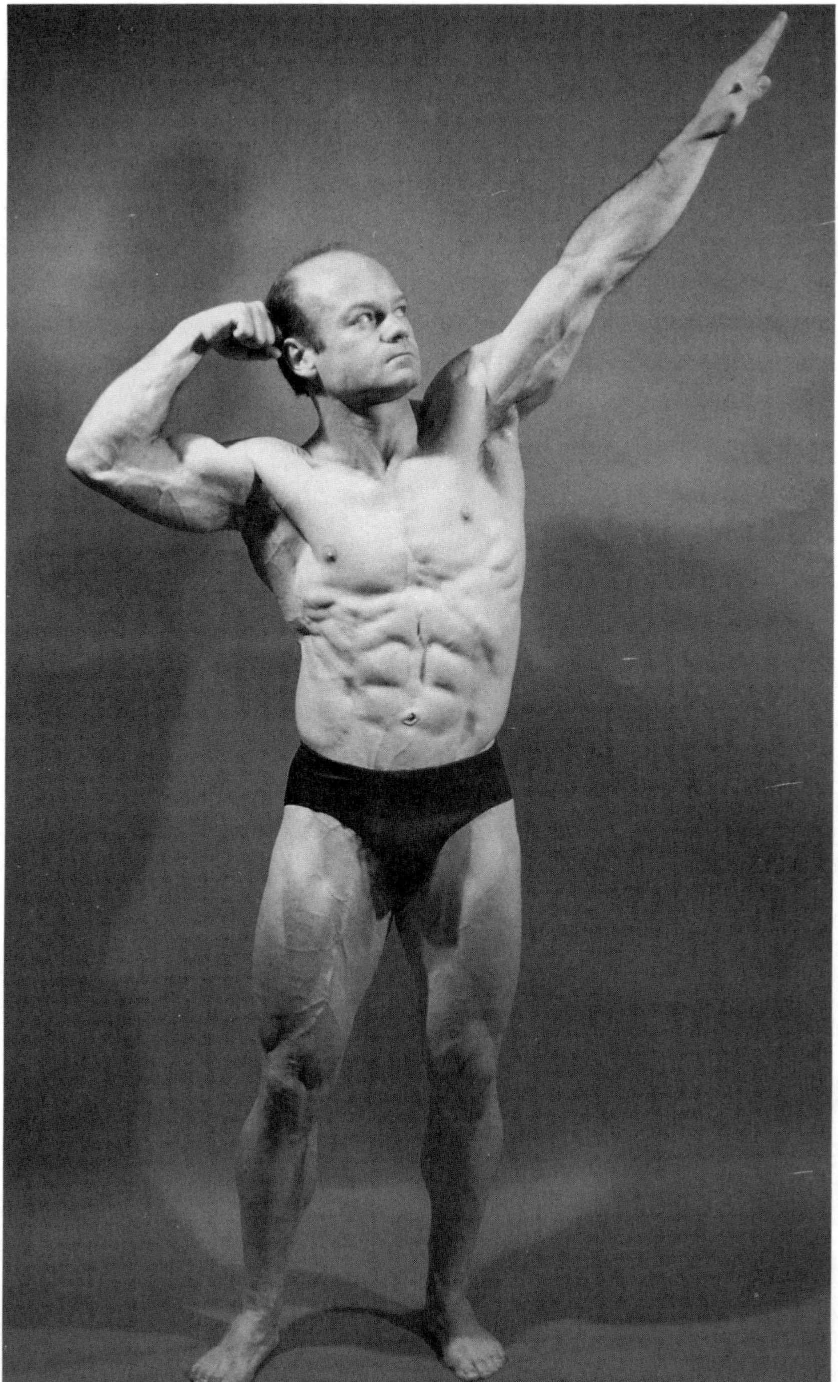

This is the first physique photo of me to appear in a muscle magazine. Peary Rader made me very happy by publishing it in *Iron Man. Photo by Bill Vollendorf.*

DIET: THE BIG PICTURE 2

THIN CALORIES

You can eat to your heart's content — if you choose thin calories instead of fat ones

Q: *I'm an 18-year-old boy who hasn't looked good his whole life. I weigh close to 225 pounds. I've been trying to lose the fat for about a year now, but I still look the same. I need help. I enclose my order for your books. Do you have any special advice for me?*

A: I understand how you feel. It's tough when you're 18 — or any age for that matter — and unhappy with the way you look. But cheer up. Things aren't as bad as they may seem.

My books will tell you how to slim down and stay that way. You'll find it's not hard once you understand what to eat and how exercise helps you lose fat. You won't have to starve yourself either. As a matter of fact, you can eat a lot once you learn what to eat and what to avoid. The details are in the books, but let's get you started with some recent findings on fat calories and some facts on thin calories as well.

As you probably know, fat makes you fat. The reason is that 1 gram of fat contains more than twice as many calories as a gram of protein or carbohydrate, 9 calories versus only 4. That's why high-fat foods such as butter, ice cream and nuts make you gain weight, while fruits and vegetables, bread and skim milk — all low-fat foods — keep you lean. But that's nothing new. You already know that. The news is that there's more to the "fat is fattening" story.

Fat Calories

Fat more important than calories

Recent research at Stanford and Harvard medical schools published in the *American Journal of Clinical Nutrition* indicates that all calories are not the same. Some calories make you fatter than others.

Harvard Medical School, after studying 141 women aged 34-59, found that the degree of excess weight was linked to fat consumption, not calorie intake. Stanford University School of Medicine came to the same conclusion. After analyzing the eating habits of 155 sedentary obese men, aged 30-59, the researchers determined that the proportion of daily calories that came from fat, not the number of calories per se, was directly linked to bodyfat percentage in the men.

Tufts University Diet & Nutrition Letter summed up the two studies: "What it comes down to is that if two men require 2,000 calories a day each, the one who eats a greater proportion of his 2,000 calories as fat is more likely to end up with bodyfat than the one who takes in more of his calories as carbohydrate." Apparently, fat calories are more easily converted to bodyfat than other calories. Here's how it works.

Experiments at the University of Massachusetts Medical School, discussed in the *University of California, Berkeley Wellness Letter,* show that dietary fat can be turned into bodyfat with just 3% of its energy used in the conversion process, while it takes 23% of calories from carbohydrate to turn it into fat stores. In other words, if you consume 100 excess carbohydrate calories, only 77 of them will end up as bodyfat; but if you consume the same number of excess calories as fat, 97 will turn up on your body as fat stores. That's a difference of 20%; over time it can make a big difference in your level of bodyfat.

The bottom line is that fat is your enemy. It makes you fat. There's a section in *The Lean Advantage 2* called "Eating the Low-Fat Way." Read it carefully. It'll help you reduce the fat calories in your diet. (You do need some fat in your diet, about 10% of your calories. Americans, on average, consume 40% of their calories as fat.)

Powerful Idea

Water plus bulk equals thin calories

That's the story on fat calories. Now let's look at thin calories, calories from foods that help you stay lean. These are foods that contain a lot of water and bulk. *Muscle & Fitness* contributor Lawrence E. Lamb, M.D., writing in *The Health Letter,* says: "A major factor in determining how many calories are in your food is how much water it contains. . . . A second factor that affects the calorie content and composition of food is bulk."

That's just common sense, isn't it? My mother used to ask my father, who was a medical doctor, what she could eat that wouldn't make her fat. He always told her to have some water. She didn't like that answer much, but there's no getting around the fact that my father was correct. Water contains no calories to make you fat.

The same is true of the bulk, fiber, in your food. Fiber contains almost no calories. It's the part of plant food that isn't digested.

This simple but powerful idea — water plus bulk equals thin calories —will help you select foods that make and keep you lean.

Examples

Stick to the Source

Processed or refined foods usually have the water and bulk removed. The farther away you get from the food source — the garden, orchard or field — the more fattening food becomes. Here's some examples.

A cup of raw grapes (153 grams) directly from the vine gives you 106 calories. But remove the water from the grapes and consume one cup (165 grams) of raisins, and you get four times as many calories, 477 versus 106. Now add sugar, lard and flour — all refined foods with the water and bulk removed — to make raisin pie, and you're really talking serious calories.

The same thing happens as you move from whole grains cooked in water, to white bread, to cake. The calories increase with each refining step, as more bulk is removed and sweeteners and fats are added.

You get the idea. Make foods with plenty of water and bulk the cornerstone of your diet. Fresh fruits and vegetables and whole grains are the foods to emphasize.

Here's my advice to you in a nutshell: Read the books carefully and remember that fat is fattening, and water and bulk are thinning. You'll be looking good soon. I guarantee it.

PYRAMID POWER

New government guidelines point to leaner diets and a leaner America

A switch from pie shape to pyramid shape could change your shape. Last year the U.S. Department of Agriculture announced a new shape for the ideal American diet — a pyramid built on a base of grain products and, equally important, narrowing at the top to show that fats and sweets should be "used sparingly." Vegetables and fruits occupy the second tier of the pyramid, indicating that they should make up a large part of a healthy diet.

Dairy and meat products occupy the next, narrower portions of the pyramid — right below fats and sweets — suggesting a need for moderation.

The pyramid replaces the familiar pie chart used since 1946 to help Americans memorize the Basic Four Food Groups: milk, meat, bread-cereal and vegetable-fruit. The change sends a powerful new message of proportionality. At a glance, the pyramid tells us to restrict fat and sugar — and eat more fruits, vegetables and, especially, grains. That's quite a different message than the now discarded food circle that emphasized variety and gave equal weight to each of the basic food groups. The old message was: About half of the diet should be dairy

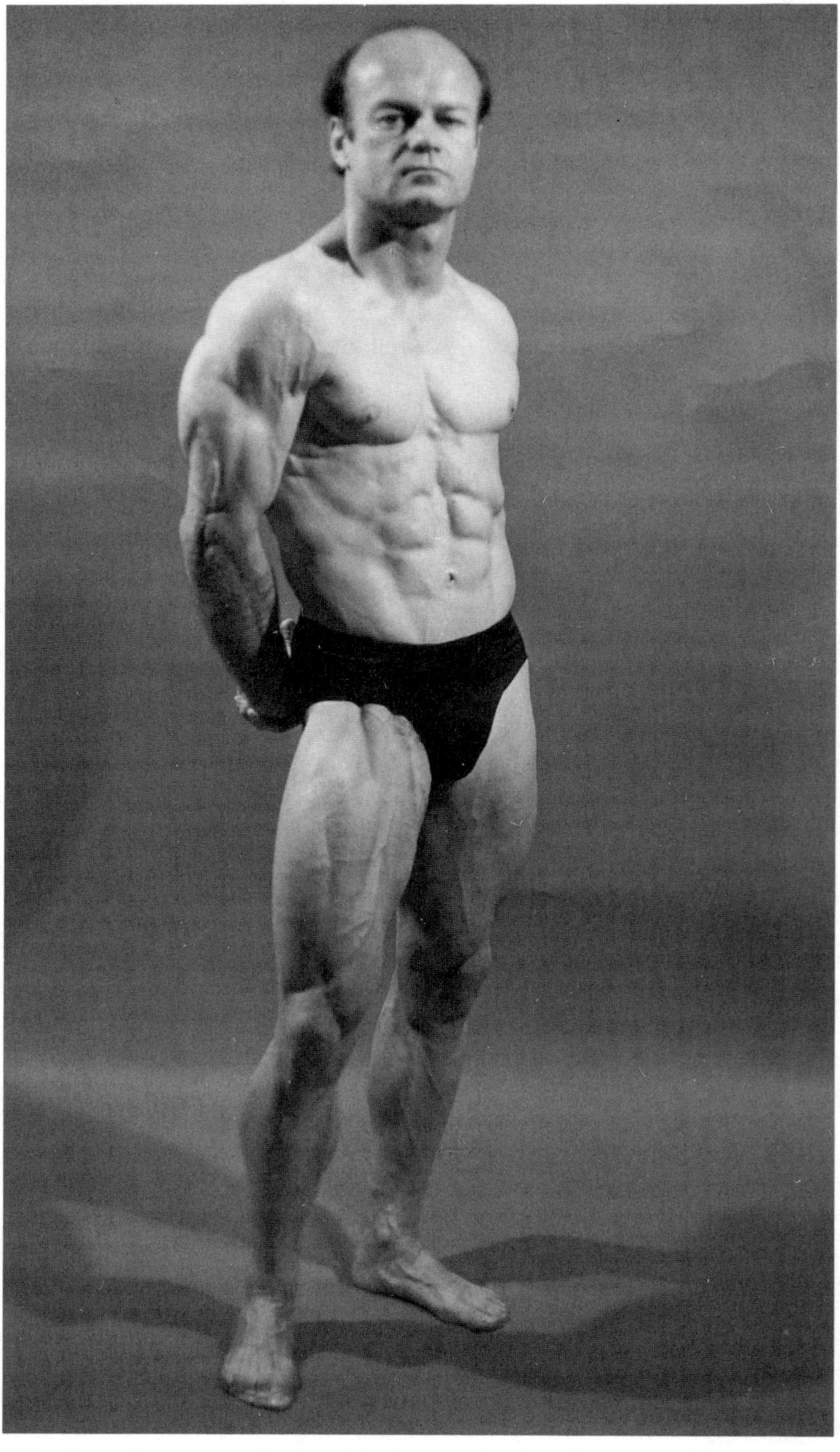

This photo also appeared in *Iron Man* in the mid-70s. *Photo by Bill Vollendorf.*

and meat products. That was rejected because it encouraged eating a diet high in animal fat and lacking in fiber.

The New Message

Bread — a new slice to dieting

The new message — eat lots of bread, cereal, rice and pasta — will surprise many. We've all heard people say, "I need to go on a diet and lose some weight; I think I'll cut down on bread and potatoes." Perhaps you've even said the same thing yourself. Well, the pyramid says loud and clear that that's the wrong approach. The truth is that bread can help you lose weight.

In my book *Lean For Life*, I included a study conducted at Michigan State University by Dr. Olaf Mickelsen, a professor of nutrition. I am going to repeat it here, because it's such a wonderful demonstration that bread is, in fact, a dieter's best friend.

Here's Mickelsen's conclusion: "Contrary to what most people think, bread in large amounts is an ideal food in a weight reducing regimen. Recent work in our laboratory indicates that slightly overweight young men lost weight in a painless and practically effortless manner when they included 12 slices of bread per day in their program. The bread was eaten with their meals. As a result, they became satisfied before they consumed their usual quota of calories. The subjects were admonished to restrict those foods that were concentrated sources of energy [that is, very high in calories]; otherwise they were free to eat as much as they desired."

Significantly, Mickelsen's charge to the students was much the same as the new nutrition-education pyramid, which recommends 6-11 servings each day from the bread group.

Mickelsen's eight-week study involved 16 young men. Eight were given a high-fiber bread; they lost an average of 19.4 pounds! The other eight were served a low-fiber bread. Their average weight loss was 13.7 pounds.

How could it be that these young men stuffed themselves with bread and lost weight? It's simple. Bread — like all starches, fruits and vegetables — fills the stomach and leaves no room for excessive calories from other foods. Plus, bread (and other bulky carbohydrate foods) makes you feel satisfied — without giving you too many calories. High-fiber bread, of course, is better than the low-fiber variety, because it provides more chewing satisfaction and takes up more room in the stomach. That's why the students eating the high-fiber bread lost more weight.

In *Eat Right* (Arco Publishing, 1979), British epidemiologist Denis Burkitt, M.D., gives the results of a similar experiment in which potatoes were consumed. Twenty-three young Irishmen were fed 2 pounds of potatoes every day for three months. They were allowed to eat anything else they wanted so long as they ate the potatoes. They also lost weight. Potatoes, of course, are bulky and high in fiber. They filled the young men up, just like the bread in Mickelsen's study, and kept their calorie consumption down.

What's On Top

The extras will kill you

It's not bread and potatoes that are fattening, it's what goes on top that adds inches to your waistline. It's not the toast, it's the butter. It's not the baked potato, it's the sour cream. It's not the salad, it's the oily dressing. That brings us to the point of the new pyramid: Fat and sugar are fattening. They are fattening because — unlike grain, vegetables and fruit — they are concentrated-calorie foods; they provide a large number of calories in a small volume.

Fat contains more calories per gram than any other kind of food. Each gram of fat contains nine calories, while 1 gram of protein or carbohydrate contains only four calories. The problem with sugar is basically the same. Sugar has a lot of calories squeezed into a small volume of food. To illustrate, 1 ounce of sugar has 109 calories, about as many calories as found in 5 ounces of bananas; and 1 pound of apples contain 242 calories, whereas 1 pound of caramel candy has 1,840. Obviously, bananas or apples fill your stomach and satisfy your appetite with fewer calories than sugar or sugar-filled candy. As I wrote in *Ripped*: "When you eat all the sugar, or all the sugar-filled foods you want, you take in more calories than your body can use and you become fat. By contrast, you can gorge yourself on apples and you won't take in more calories than your body can use and you won't become fat."

To make matters even worse, fat and sugar stimulate your appetite; they encourage you to overeat because they taste good. Ask yourself: Would I be inclined to eat more baked potato with sour cream or without? Would I eat more baked apple sprinkled with brown sugar or plain?

It boils down to this: Eat a diet made up largely of grains, fruits and vegetables — and avoid foods high in fat and sugar — and you can eat almost as much as you want and still lose weight. You'll actually find it hard to overeat. What happens is that you become full and satisfied before you take in more calories than you burn. So, here's to pyramid power. The government's new food chart is a winner. Combined with a program of regular exercise — weights and aerobics — it shows the way to a leaner body and better health.

YOUR MUSCLES' APPETITE

New research emphasizes a special need for protein

About 10 years ago, I wrote a column highlighting research suggesting that the RDA (Recommended Dietary Allowance) for protein may be inadequate for physically active individuals. Research at that time showed that protein, especially the amino acid leucine, provided a significant portion of the total calories used during exercise. This was important news because it challenged the conventional view that exercise did not increase the need for dietary protein. The bodybuilder's gut feeling that he or she needed more protein was proving to be correct. My guess at that time was that bodybuilders need a little more than 1 gram of protein per 2.2 pounds (1 kilogram) of bodyweight. It now appears that I was a little short of the mark.

Mark Tarnopolsky, Ph.D., one of the most active researchers on the optimal levels of protein for active people, summarized the latest research in *The Physician and Sportsmedicine* (March 1993). It turns out that hard-training athletes may actually need twice as much protein as an inactive person. The need and manner of use varies, based on the type of exercise. Significantly, if you work hard at both strength and endurance training, your protein needs may be the greatest of all athletes.

According to Tarnopolsky, endurance exercise increases amino acid oxidation, while resistance exercise speeds protein turnover and muscle protein synthesis. As explained in my earlier column, endurance exercise has been clearly shown to speed the oxidation of the essential amino acid leucine for energy; the more intense the exercise, the more leucine is burned. That, of course, means endurance athletes need additional protein for normal building and repair purposes. Strength training also uses protein, but in a different way. While it does not increase amino acid oxidation, resistance exercise increases whole-body protein turnover and muscle protein synthesis or formation. As Tarnopolsky observes, that's not surprising given the obvious fact that weight training promotes muscle growth.

Specific Protein Requirements

U.S. Recommended Daily Allowance inadequate

Nitrogen balance testing, which measures the protein entering and leaving the body, shows that the U.S. Recommended Daily Allowance for protein — 0.8 gram of protein per 2.2 pounds of bodyweight — is inadequate for most athletes. Well-controlled studies using this method estimate that the protein requirement for endurance athletes is 1.2-1.6 grams/kilogram/day. The higher estimates are for very elite endurance athletes. The range is about the same for bodybuilders. Tarnopolsky and colleagues have found that elite bodybuilders doing maintenance training require about 1.2 g/kg/day, while bodybuilders training with increasing intensity use about 1.62 g/kg/day.

And finally, to me, the most interesting discovery: "Resistance athletes performing high-intensity power sports (e.g., football, rugby) in addition to circuit weight training require about 1.76 g/kg/day." Clearly bodybuilders like me, who alternate high-intensity aerobics with high-intensity weight training, fall in that category. Apparently, we have the greatest need for protein. When you think about it, that makes sense. People doing balanced training — strength and endurance — are burning extra amino acids during aerobic sessions and, in addition, increasing protein turnover and synthesis in weight workouts.

What about women? Does gender have an effect on protein requirements? Tarnopolsky says that nitrogen balance tests show that female endurance athletes require about 25% less protein than men. Female bodybuilders probably need more protein than that, because they have more muscle than other female athletes.

No Problem

Athletes can easily meet protein needs

Computer analysis of my diet by the Cooper Aerobics Center in Dallas shows that even a person on a near-vegetarian diet can easily meet the newly discovered protein requirements for athletes. Tarnopolsky says, assuming their energy intake is adequate, that most athletes will fulfill their enlarged protein requirement by simply taking care to consume at least 10% of their daily calories in the form of protein.

Using a three-day food record, two weekdays and one weekend day, the Cooper Center determined that my diet is 18% protein, almost twice what Tarnopolsky says I need. (The balance of my diet is 65% complex carbohydrates, 14% fat and 3% sugar.) That's true even though I consume only an ounce or two of lean beef or chicken each day. Most of my high-quality protein comes from skimmed milk and nonfat yogurt. I eat only an occasional egg. My other protein comes from foods that individually do not contain all the essential amino acids, but when eaten in combination do provide complete protein: cereal, bread, nut butter, potatoes and high-protein vegetables such as broccoli. Even the orange I slice over my morning cereal contains more than a gram of protein.

In the light of the recent findings, I'm glad that I've always attended to my protein needs. From the time I took up weight training as a teenager, I've taken care to include some high-quality protein (milk, eggs or meat) with every meal. Needless to say, I've also consumed my share of protein supplements. Thanks to the teaching of far-sighted pioneers like Bob Hoffman and Joe Weider, I've always consumed adequate protein.

Take care to do the same — especially if you're on an energy-restricted diet. Still, don't lose sight of the fact that excess calories from any source — carbohydrate, fat or protein — build fat, not muscle. Eat a balanced diet and don't overeat.

CHAPTER THREE

FOCUS ON SPECIFIC FOODS

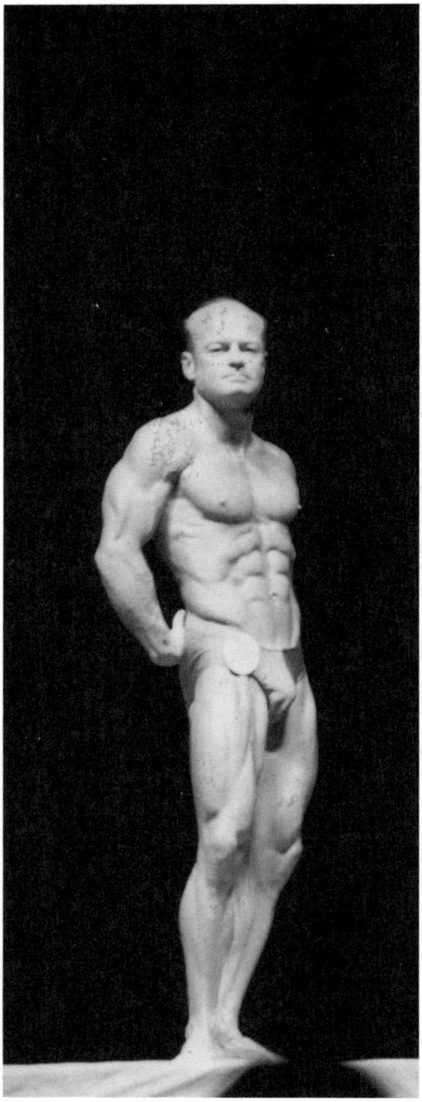

This was taken at one of my first physique contests, the 1978 Mr. New Mexico. I won the Most Muscular Man award and Best legs. *Photo by Bruce Bambrook.*

FOCUS ON SPECIFIC FOODS 3

WHAT ABOUT WATER?

Q: *I haven't seen anything in your books about water. Is it all right to drink as much water as I want throughout the day, or will it smooth me out?*

A: You're worried that water might smooth you out. Others write because they've heard that proper water intake is the key to weight loss. Actually, there's some truth in both extremes, but in the main both concerns are unfounded. Water is, nevertheless, a very important nutrient.

Our bodies are about two-thirds water — 55-65% water for females, 65-75% water for males. A woman's body contains less water because she has more fat and fat holds less water than lean tissue. Muscle is about 75% water. Obviously, water is very important to our wellbeing.

Vital Nutrient

In fact, nutritionists often say water is our most vital nutrient. It carries food and oxygen to cells and removes waste products. Water is essential to the digestive as well as the elimination process. It lubricates our joints and, through perspiration, keeps us cool. Our bodies simply can't function properly without water. You can live a long time without food, but two or three days without water and you're a goner.

In her recent television special, Rachel McLish (who looked spectacular) said she drinks several glasses of water first thing every morning. That's not a bad idea. Most of us don't drink enough water.

Thirst is an imperfect signal. You should drink at least six — preferably eight — eight-ounce glasses of water a day. Coffee and tea are not good substitutes, however, because they are mild diuretics, causing the kidneys to be more active and excrete more water than they would otherwise.

Keep in mind that the food we eat contains water. Even meat and bread are one-half and one-third water, respectively. As you know from reading my books, I recommend eating (besides whole grains) lots of fresh fruits and vegetables, which are two-thirds or more water. So on this kind of diet you consume plenty of water without forcing liquids.

I know what you're thinking at this point. You've read that bodybuilders sometimes have a water retention problem that makes them look smooth. This is quite true. The cause, however, is sodium, not water per se. You'll find a complete discussion of the sodium factor in my book *Ripped 2*. Briefly, sodium (as in salt) tends to concentrate in the fluids surrounding the cells. Taking in excess sodium causes an accumulation of sodium outside the cell and pulls water from the cell into the space between the cells. This creates a puffy and bloated appearance. The solution is not to cut back on water, but to select foods low in sodium. That's really pretty easy, because unprocessed, natural foods are generally low in sodium.

And, believe it or not, the way to get rid of water retention is to drink more water. Leroy R. Perry, Jr., the chiropractic physician famous for treating worldclass athletes, pointed this out recently in *Parade* magazine: "If you're not drinking enough water, your body starts retaining water to compensate for this shortage," he said. "So paradoxical as it may seem, the way to eliminate fluid retention is to drink *more* water, not less."

Drink To Lose?

What about those who say that proper water intake is the key to weight loss? As I mentioned earlier, there's some truth in that, but water certainly won't wash fat away by itself. Losing weight still comes back to calorie output exceeding calorie input. The famous water diets don't work — that is, unless they also create a negative calorie balance.

Lawrence E. Lamb, MD, in his book *The Weighting Game* (Lyle Stuart, 1988), doesn't mince words. "Drinking lots of water or fluids will not affect your fat stores," he states emphatically.

Preventative medicine specialist Arno L. Jensen, MD of the Cooper Clinic in Dallas, agrees. "There's no metabolic magic in water," he says. Jensen, of course, points out that the water has no calories and it can be helpful to the extent that it leaves no room in the stomach for calorie-containing foods. Lamb adds that extra liquids cause the colon to empty sooner.

That's where the water diets have validity. Water makes your bowels function better. In fact, high-fiber foods and water are the best treatment for constipation. Plus, as I've already said, drinking water helps get rid of excess water in the tissues.

To the extent that it helps to eliminate fluid retention and constipation, water is an aid to the fat-loss process. The benefit is mostly psychological, however. That's because water retention and constipation prevent fat-loss from registering on your scales. If you are constipated or retaining water, your weight may go up when in fact you're losing fat. This is discouraging and might well cause a person to give up on his or her fat-reduction program. So, to the extent that drinking extra water makes the results of a sensible weight-loss program more apparent, it is a benefit.

By all means, drink as much water as you want throughout the day. I encourage you to drink more water than you need to quench your thirst. Drinking water definitely will not make you smooth. What's more, it will help your body function efficiently and make it easier to monitor true changes in bodyfat level.

A BAD BREAK FOR EGGS?

They're high in cholesterol, but there's more to the story

Q: *I've just read in your first book,* Ripped, *that you ate 12-18 eggs a day when you were preparing for the Past-40 Mr. America contest. Obviously, the diet worked because you won the short class. Do you recommend that people eat a dozen or more eggs a day to get ripped? What about the cholesterol in eggs?*

A: Next to questions about my peanut butter lunch, probably the thing I've been asked about most over the years is all those eggs I ate in 1978. First, I want to state emphatically that I do not recommend that anybody eat a dozen or more eggs a day!

One reason *Ripped* is still a best seller — it's now in its eighth printing — is that I let it all hang out, so to speak. In *Ripped,* I tell what I did wrong as well as what I did right. Eating a dozen or more eggs a day as a part of a low-carb, high-protein diet is one of the mistakes I made while wrestling my way through the maze of diets in vogue at the time.

In the '70s, many bodybuilders used a low-carb, high-protein, high-fat diet to cut up for competition. Interestingly, that diet may now be attempting a comeback. As you may have noticed, there's recently been a spate of articles in the bodybuilding press touting the high-fat diet as a way to increase muscle gain. As you read further on in *Ripped,* you'll find that I abandoned that diet the next year as I prepared for the 1979 Past-40 Mr. USA (I won my class again and the Most Muscular Man award). The reason was simple: That diet made me feel tired and awful. Without the carbohydrates my brain needed to function, I couldn't think — or train — properly. "If your body and your brain can't function properly on a low-carbohydrate diet," I wrote in *Ripped,* "then the low-carbohydrate diet can't be the best diet for achievement of maximum muscle and minimum fat."

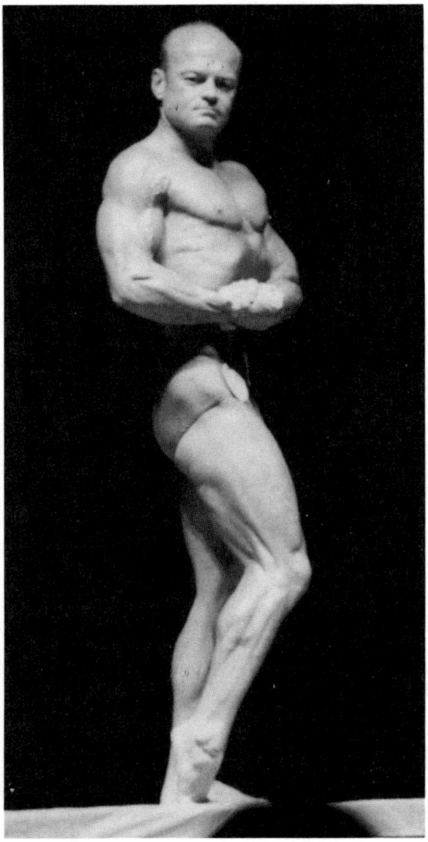

Another photo taken at the 1978 Mr. New Mexico contest. *Photo by Bruce Bambrook.*

Late in 1978, I said, "No," to the low-carb, high-fat diet and went back to a balanced diet of natural foods. The body-composition test results contained in the final chapters of *Ripped* prove that was the correct decision. On the low-carb diet I experienced every bodybuilder's nightmare: I lost more muscle — almost twice as much — than fat. On a balanced diet, however, I reversed the trend. I not only felt better, I lost more fat than muscle. Since then, I haven't looked back. And believe me, I'll never again eat a dozen or more eggs a day.

Nevertheless, I must tell you that my blood cholesterol level did not increase when I was eating 18 eggs a day. Several years before, I had tried to reduce my blood cholesterol by going on a low-cholesterol diet. My cholesterol went down for a while, but it soon returned to its previous level. That's because the biggest source of cholesterol is not in the food you eat, but in the cholesterol that is manufactured by your own body, mostly the liver. In 1978 when I ate all those eggs, my liver apparently compensated in the opposite direction.

Your Body Makes Cholesterol

There's more there than you think

According to the well-respected *Health Letter* edited by *M&F* columnist Lawrence E. Lamb, MD, the normal adult liver manufactures 1,500-2,500 mg of cholesterol a day. In addition, the cholesterol in the lining of your small intestine, which is constantly being shed, provides another 500 mg of cholesterol. The average American diet contains 450-700 mg. That means, according to Lamb, the average American's intestine contains a combined total of 3,000-7,000 mg of cholesterol a day. Cholesterol is absorbed into your circulation from this total pool of cholesterol, not just from the cholesterol in your diet.

As you obviously know, eggs are notoriously high in cholesterol. Many doctors say that we should not exceed 300 mg of cholesterol per day. One egg contains more than 200 mg. So my diet in 1978 contains an excess of the recommended allotment of cholesterol. As already indicated, my liver apparently adjusted by cutting back on the amount of cholesterol manufactured.

You may not be so lucky, however. According to Lamb, genes play an important role in determining cholesterol levels. Some people are genetically predisposed to high total cholesterol levels — and high rates of heart attacks and strokes — while others have good genes that allow them to consume high amounts of fat and cholesterol and still maintain low levels of cholesterol in their blood.

In addition, my high activity level and relatively low total calorie intake in 1978 probably played a role in keeping my cholesterol level in check. It's important to understand that cholesterol is not a fat. It's an inert alcohol that can't be broken down to release calories. While eggs are indeed high in cholesterol, one large egg contains only 82 calories and about 6 grams of total fat. In spite of my high egg consumption, my total calorie intake was relatively low, especially considering my high activity level.

Again, it is not just the cholesterol in your diet that's important. As Lamb points out in *The Health Letter,* the most common cause for undesirable cholesterol levels is lifestyle: specifically consuming too many calories, too much fat and not getting enough exercise. Too much fat, especially saturated fat, will cause your liver to produce more cholesterol than you are likely to get in your diet. Plus, exercise increases HDL cholesterol, the good lipoprotein, which clears the cholesterol out of your cells and arteries.

The Lifestyle/Cholesterol Connection

High activity might lower cholesterol

The Paleolithic Prescription (Harper & Row, 1988), the brilliant book by a team of doctors and anthropologists about the lifestyle of ancient man, contains further evidence that it is not just the cholesterol in your diet that is important. According to authors S. Boyd Eaton, MD, Marjorie Shostak and Melvin Konner, MD, Ph.D., paleolithic humans, because of their heavy reliance on meat, consumed up to 1,000 mg of cholesterol a day, more than three times the currently recommended amount.

"Recent hunters and gatherers, with diets (and general life-styles) resembling those of late paleolithic humans, have extremely low serum cholesterol levels despite their high levels of dietary cholesterol," write the authors. For example, the Masai, lion-hunting pastoralists who live along the Kenya-Tanzania border in Africa, consume from 600-2000 mg of cholesterol a day, yet their serum cholesterol levels remain low, generally ranging from 115-145 mg. Clearly, factors other than the total amount of cholesterol in their food are at work. Their example, say Eaton and his colleagues, adds to the evidence that dietary cholesterol, by itself, has a relatively limited influence on serum cholesterol levels.

A 1987 study of South African egg farm workers described in *The Paleolithic Prescription* is even more to the point of your question. These workers, naturally, eat a great number of eggs. Nevertheless, because fat provides only 20% of their daily calories (versus 40% for the average American), their serum cholesterol levels average 180 mg — higher than most doctors would like but still significantly lower than those of most Americans.

I was lucky. My excessive egg consumption in 1978 doesn't seem to have had any ill effects. Be that as it may, I rarely eat eggs now. Most doctors recommend limiting egg consumption, and I believe that's the wise course — for bodybuilders and others.

DON'T GET JUICED

Bulk is what's missing when you get trendy

Q: *I would like to lose about 10 pounds, and I have a question for you on diet. You recommend eating lots of fresh fruits and vegetables. As you know, many claims are being made for juicing these days. I understand that over two million juicing machines were sold in the United States last year. Will juicing help me lose fat? I now drink eight ounces of organically grown juice with breakfast each morning.*

A: I do indeed recommend that people eat lots of whole fruits and vegetables (and whole grains) to become and stay lean. Not only do these foods provide many of the vitamins and minerals we need to stay healthy, they are also filling and satisfying. They fill you up without filling you out, so to speak. Unfortunately, that benefit is reduced when fruits and vegetables are made into juice. Whatever the health benefits of juicing — some of the claims are questionable and made without supporting evidence —juicing is no help to a dieter. It's actually counterproductive.

Most juicers extract the juice from the produce and leave behind the bulky pulp. That's a drawback because the pulp contains significant amounts of vitamins and minerals. It also contains lots of fiber, and most Americans — especially those trying to lose weight — need more fiber. Fiber keeps you lean. It's a dieter's best friend. That's because it contains almost no calories. It's the part of the plant food that isn't digested. It passes through the digestive system virtually unchanged. Significantly, it helps fill up your stomach before you get too many calories.

That's why in *Ripped* I counseled: "Avoid fruit or vegetable juices because all the natural fiber and bulk have been removed. This increases the calorie concentration. Eat the fruits or vegetables instead."

For example, it takes a full pound of oranges — that's about three average oranges — to make 6-8 ounces of juice. Ask yourself: Which would be more filling and satisfying, three whole oranges or one cup of orange juice?

British Apple Study

Whole fruit more satisfying than processed

Now let me tell you about a study that explains what actually happens when we alter foods by removing the fiber and bulk and, therefore, increase the calorie density. The study involves apples and was performed at the Royal Infirmary in Bristol, England.

The following description of the study appeared in Jane Brody's *Nutrition Book* (W.W. Norton 1981): "Ten healthy people were given test 'meals' of either whole apples, pureed apples (applesauce) or apple juice. Each meal contained the same amount of sugar. It took 17 minutes to eat the apples, six minutes to down the puree and 1½ minutes to drink the juice. It should come as no surprise to learn that the individuals reported greater satisfaction after eating the apples than after drinking the juice, with the puree providing an intermediate level of satiety."

Importantly, this experiment went beyond the subjective feelings of the test subjects. The researchers actually recorded changes in blood sugar and insulin levels to determine if there was a physiological basis for the different degrees of hunger satisfaction.

"Blood sugar rose to similar levels after all three meals," Brody reported, "but the insulin level of the blood rose twice as high after the juice than after the whole apple. One to three hours later, the blood sugar levels dropped — back to normal after the apples, but to a level distinctly below normal after the juice. An intermediate but below-

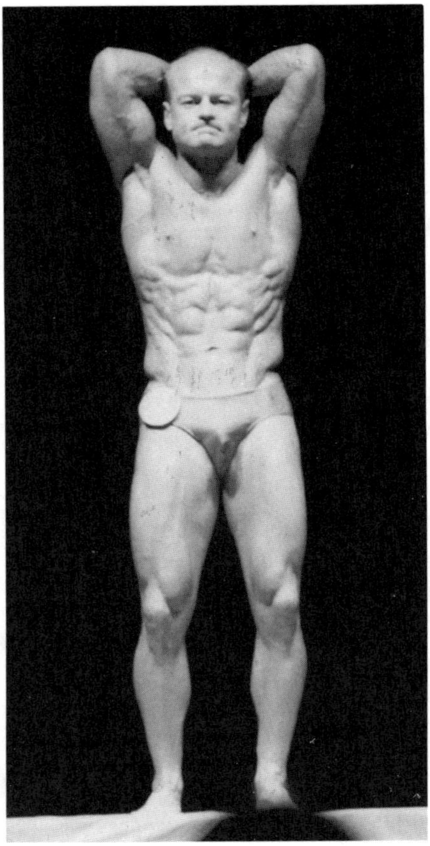

Photo by Bruce Bambrook.

normal blood sugar level occurred after the puree."

Commenting on the significance of the different blood sugar and insulin levels in the three groups, Brody wrote: "These below normal levels [of blood sugar], called rebound hypoglycemia, are usually associated with feelings of hunger. Thus, the fiber in the whole apples reduced the demand for insulin and produced a longer lasting feeling of satiety." In other words whole apples produced long-term hunger satisfaction. In contrast, apple juice and applesauce, both concentrated calorie foods, caused low blood sugar and only short-term satisfaction; soon after eating them you're hungry again.

So you see, juicing is a step in the wrong direction for dieters. It provides food in a more concentrated form, which means it takes more calories to make you feel full. It deprives you of the satisfaction of chewing. It is downed so fast that your normal appetite control mechanism has no time to register when you've had enough. Plus, as the British apple study demonstrated, it promotes rebound hypoglycemia and only short-term hunger satisfaction.

I suggest you have juice as an occasional treat, rather than every morning. Nothing tastes better than a cold glass of orange juice on a hot summer day, and it's certainly better for you than soda pop. But for everyday consumption — especially if you're trying to lose fat — here's the bottom line on juicing from the September 1992 *Consumer Reports on Health*: "There's no juice that's better than the produce itself."

GLYCOGEN REFILL

Carbohydrate-rich foods load your muscle fuel storage tanks

During a visit to California about 14 years ago, I had a postworkout meal with a well-known professional bodybuilder. My friend was preparing for a competition, and he'd just finished a hard training session. When we arrived at his apartment, his girlfriend had lunch ready for us: sauteed chicken breasts. That's it, chicken breasts.

Frankly, I enjoyed the simple meal, but I knew it was the wrong thing to eat after a workout. As I wrote in *Ripped,* "Your body and your brain can't function properly on a low carbohydrate diet." Many bodybuilders at that time, however, believed they would gain fat if they ate carbs after training.

I thought that idea was now passé — until I flicked on the TV a few days ago to catch the last few minutes of a nationally syndicated workout show. I was just in time to hear the star sign off with this tip for viewers: "Remember," he said, "after a workout, what your muscles need is protein. Egg whites are good." And almost as an afterthought, he added, "Have some rice too."

It's true, bodybuilders and other hard-training athletes need protein for repair and growth. Nevertheless, the single most important nutrient in an active person's diet is carbohydrate. Carbohydrates are the predominant source of energy for exercising muscles — especially after intense training.

Carbohydrates & Performance

Proof of a direct link

As Dr. George Sheehan states in his latest book, *Running To Win* (Rodale 1992), there's a direct relationship between carbohydrate consumption and performance. That's important for construction workers and housewives — or anyone else who does hard physical work — but it's also crucial for someone doing high-intensity training.

It's long been known that eating a higher-than-usual amount of carbohydrate enhances endurance. Distance runners for some years have been carbo loading to improve their performances. More recently, however, we've learned that short, hard training sessions — like those of bodybuilders, who often perform six or more workouts a week — reduce muscle glycogen considerably. According to the February 1993 issue of *The Physician and Sportsmedicine,* muscle glycogen can be depleted after only a 15-30-minute exercise session performed at very high intensities. "Athletes who attempt to train daily at intensities that deplete muscle glycogen must take extraordinary measures to eat carbohydrates at optimal times," says the journal.

When muscle glycogen is depleted, you are forced to lower the intensity of your workouts. Runners call it "hitting the wall." Even a one-hour run can reduce muscle glycogen considerably. If glycogen isn't replaced over time, the runner will develop fatigue and perform poorly.

For bodybuilders and other strength athletes the results are equally devastating. A bodybuilder's progress depends on his or her ability to train hard; intensity is the key factor in building strength and muscle size. What's more, your brain relies on carbohydrates to function properly. The energy for your brain comes first from the carbohydrate (glucose) contained in your circulating blood, and then from the carbohydrates stores in your liver. According to Lawrence Lamb, MD, the glucose that's circulating in your blood and stored in your liver is enough to tide your brain over during the night, but that's about it. People who deprive themselves of carbohydrate simply cannot think or train properly.

Specific Recommendations

How & When?

Most nutritionists agree that athletes should obtain about 70% of their total caloric intake from carbohydrate. But there's more to it than that. Timing is important as well. The two hours immediately after training are especially critical. The problem is that muscle glycogen is normally resynthesized at a rate of only 5% per hour. Even when diet is ideal, approximately 20 hours are required to recover muscle glycogen stores. The one exception is the two hours immediately after exercise. During that time, says *The Physician and Sportsmedicine,* muscle glycogen can be restored at the rate of 7-8% per hour. As you can see, both rates are slow. That means an active person must pay careful attention to carbohydrate intake to ensure recovery before the next workout.

Both the amount and timing of carbohydrate consumption are important. According to *The Physician and Sportsmedicine,* muscle glycogen restoration is near maximum when a 154-pound athlete consumes at least 50 grams of carbohydrate every two hours. To give you an idea how much that is, 3½ slices of bread, three oranges or one baked potato contain about 50 grams of carbohydrate. (People who weigh more or less than 154 pounds need to adjust their carbohydrate intake accordingly.) Importantly, glycogen restoration is slowed to only 2% per hour when carbohydrate intake is reduced to 25 grams every two hours.

To take full advantage of your increased capacity to restore muscle glycogen after exercise, eat foods containing more concentrated carbohydrate and less bulk. That's the opposite of the cereals, grains, fruits and vegetables I usually recommend for staying lean. The window of opportunity immediately following exercise is an exception.

You probably won't be hungry right after you exercise, so you'll want something that tastes good and is packed with nutrition. One of the many nutritious energy bars available in health-food stores and the nutrition section in supermarkets is a good place to start. Check the label. Look for something high in carbohydrates and low in fat. Fat slows digestion and blunts carbohydrate absorption. Regular candy bars are a bad choice because they usually contain lots of fat and too many calories.

In case you're wondering, it's not necessary to eat every two hours around the clock. Dr. David Costill and his colleagues at Ball State University in Muncie, Indiana have found that muscle glycogen synthesis is about the same whether carbohydrates are eaten in two large meals or seven smaller meals. The important point is to consume carbohydrates as soon as possible after training, and then eat an additional 50 grams of carbohydrate every two hours until your next large meal. After the critical postexercise period, go back to the bulky, filling, low-calorie foods that keep your energy up and your bodyfat down.

Remember, after a workout your muscles need carbohydrate — not chicken breasts or egg whites — and pronto.

CHAPTER FOUR

TIPS ON SUCCESSFUL DIETING

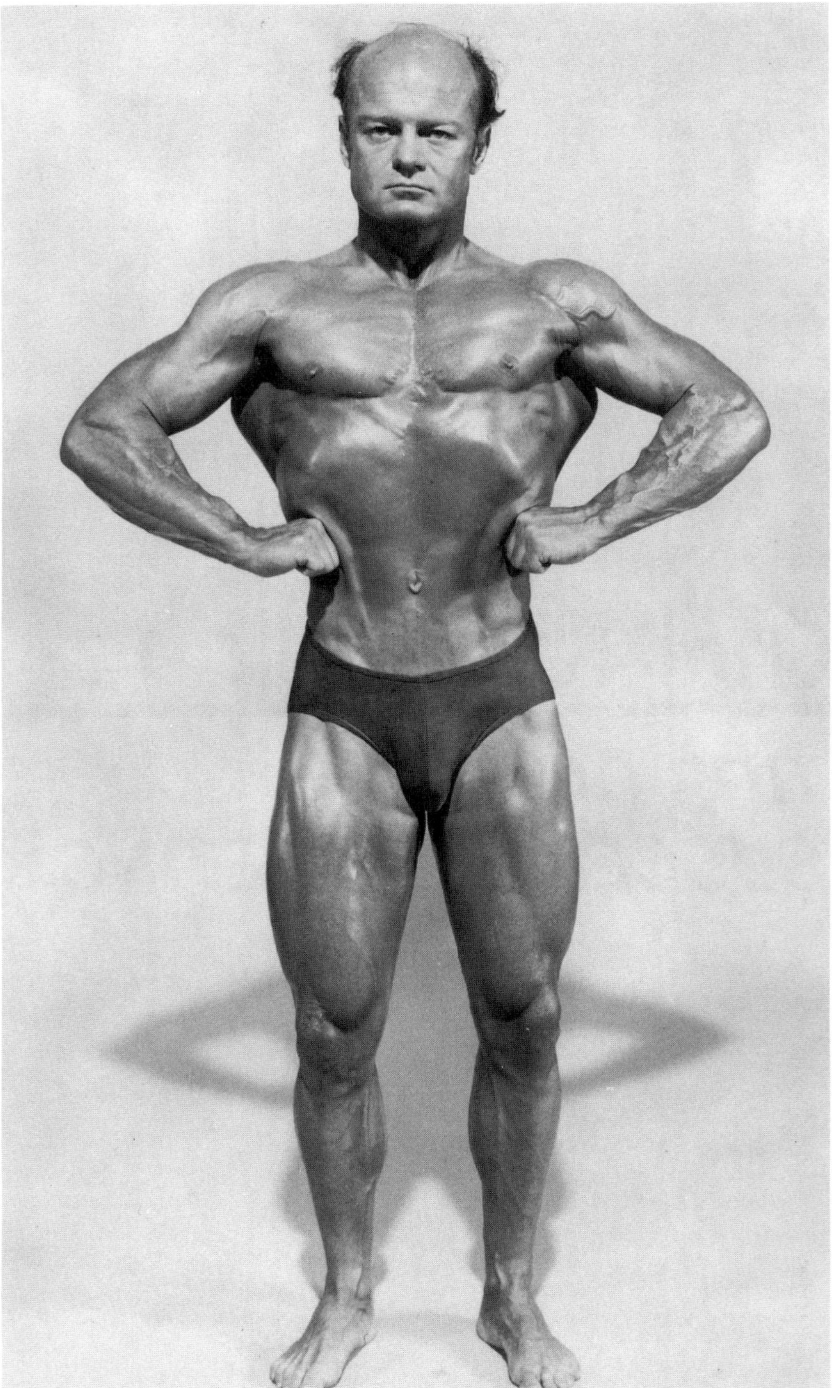

Taken backstage at the 1978 Past-40 Mr. America, where I won the short class.
Photo by Dave Sauer.

TIPS ON SUCCESSFUL DIETING 4

NEVER STAY HUNGRY

No diet based on denial works very long

A famous bodybuilder interviewed recently said he doesn't like dieting because of what it does to the individual's personality. He went on to explain: "People wonder why I get fat in the off-season. I get fat in the off-season for one particular reason: I'm happier."

I did a double take on that quote because it speaks volumes about dieters and dieting. It explains, in large part, the results of a study by Dr. Thomas Wadden at the University of Pennsylvania: Ninety-eight percent of all dieters regain their lost weight within five years.

Dieting doesn't work because it makes people unhappy; they feel hungry and deprived. As I said in *Ripped 3:* "There's a strong psychological component to eating. It's human nature to crave what you can't have, and craving usually spells doom for dieters."

Most of us have had the experience of going on an eating binge after a period of dietary deprivation. A few years ago, I clamped down on my fluid intake to solve a water retention problem I was having before a photo session.

Just knowing I couldn't drink freely made me thirsty. The problem was mainly in my mind, because I didn't dehydrate enough to cause any physical problems. It was just a matter of wanting what I couldn't have.

The result was a good illustration of what happens when you deny yourself nourishment. I went on an eating and drinking binge that lasted more than a month. I gained almost 12 pounds of fat and water, ending up at my highest bodyweight in years!

I'm certain the same psychological dynamics go on in the head of the famous bodybuilder quoted above. He makes himself miserable dieting for the big contest, and then to compensate binges and gets fat in the off-season. Unfortunately, that's the pattern most dieters follow.

Fast & Binge Roller Coaster

My friend Eric Brotman recently sent me an article from *The New York Times* about dieters and their cravings. This piece gave several hard-hitting examples of what it describes as "the fast-and-binge roller coaster." The one I liked best is bizarre, but it illustrates the intense psychological pressure that can build up during the course of a severe diet.

The story was about a 47-year-old Manhattan lawyer who had lost 143 pounds on a liquid formula diet. After a time, he started dreaming about food, and finally closed his office door one Friday, drew up an itinerary and hired a car and driver for the next day. According to *The New York Times,* from noon to 7:30 p.m. the next day, he sat in the back seat, eating. After 22 stops, surrounded by wrappers and carry-out food containers, he had consumed about 7,000 calories. (That might seem low, but it's the figure given.) He ended up gaining 21 pounds in 13 days.

This poor man's plight shows that crash diets, like those followed by many determined bodybuilders, almost always fail. The truth is that no diet based on denial and deprivation works for very long.

The One Diet That Works

The only diet that will make you lean and *keep you lean* is one that is filling and satisfying without giving you too many calories. Does such a diet exist? A study at the University of Alabama, cited by Roy Walford, MD in his book *The 120 Year Diet* (Simon & Schuster, 1987), proves that it does.

Two groups of volunteers were allowed to eat all they wanted. But one group ate only whole foods — fruit, hot cereals, skimmed milk, soups, salads, fish, chicken, rice, vegetables and whole-wheat toast and rolls. The other group ate refined foods. The refined foods included bacon, eggs, juice, buttered toast, fast foods, fried foods, roast or steak, buttered vegetables, whole milk, cake and ice cream. The whole-food eaters achieved full satisfaction from as little as 1,500 calories a day, but it took 3,000 calories of refined and processed foods to satisfy the other group.

In a letter to me Walford observed that the diet on which the University of Alabama volunteers felt satisfied closely parallels the diet described in my *Ripped* books. Needless to say, Walford, a professor of pathology at the University of California at Los Angeles School of Medicine and one of the world's leading experts on aging, recommends the whole-food diet for longevity and leanness.

So take it from Walford and me: You can be both happy *and* ripped. Moreover, if you're not happy you won't be ripped for long. The secret is not how much, but *what* you eat.

The message is clear: If lifetime leanness is your goal, "stay hungry" is the wrong slogan. To paraphrase the man in the White House, "Read my lips, never stay hungry!"

THE OWNERSHIP PRINCIPLE

The common link in diets that work

"I do not believe the human body is built to lift weight for sets and repetitions as is done when bodybuilding." That's an opinion expressed to me recently by a 50-year-old Swedish health and fitness enthusiast. Of course, I disagree and at first I paid no attention to him. Upon reflection, however, I decided that an important lesson was to be learned from him.

This Swede is no kook. He has had the same job for the last 25 years, working from midnight to around 7 a.m. He's been an observer of bodybuilding for almost as long. About 20 years ago, he bought Joe Weider's bodybuilding course and started training. Enclosed with his letter was a picture of himself holding a current issue of *Muscle & Fitness,* which showed that he's still interested in the iron game. He's followed the careers of bodybuilding greats like Bill Pearl. And he read my first book *Ripped* when it was serialized in *Bodybuilding Monthly,* a British publication. So, apparently, his opinions are formed over time, and only after long study.

After a year of lifting, he says, his blood pressure went up. Also, he sent me a picture of the scar to show that he got a hernia from deadlifting. The hernia seems to be what persuaded him that the human body — or at least *his* body — is not built to lift weights. He stopped lifting, but he didn't lose interest in health and fitness — not by a long shot. The muscles he built with weights are all gone now, he says, but his photo shows a very lean and fit 50-year-old. That's no accident.

Simple Exercise Program

He has continued to work out following a program of simple gymnastics — push-ups, sit-ups, lunges, neck bridges, one-legged squats and the like — developed by Swedish fitness adviser Arne Tammer. In addition, rain or shine, he runs/jogs around a schoolyard for 15 minutes ("no more, no less") twice a week. He runs in the clothes he has on, "even if it's boots and a raincoat." Like I said, he's no casual fitness buff.

His father died at 53 of a heart attack, and it's clear he wants to avoid a similar fate. That's why he never eats meat and doesn't drink milk. Seven days a week, he eats only fish, potatoes, rice, tomatoes,

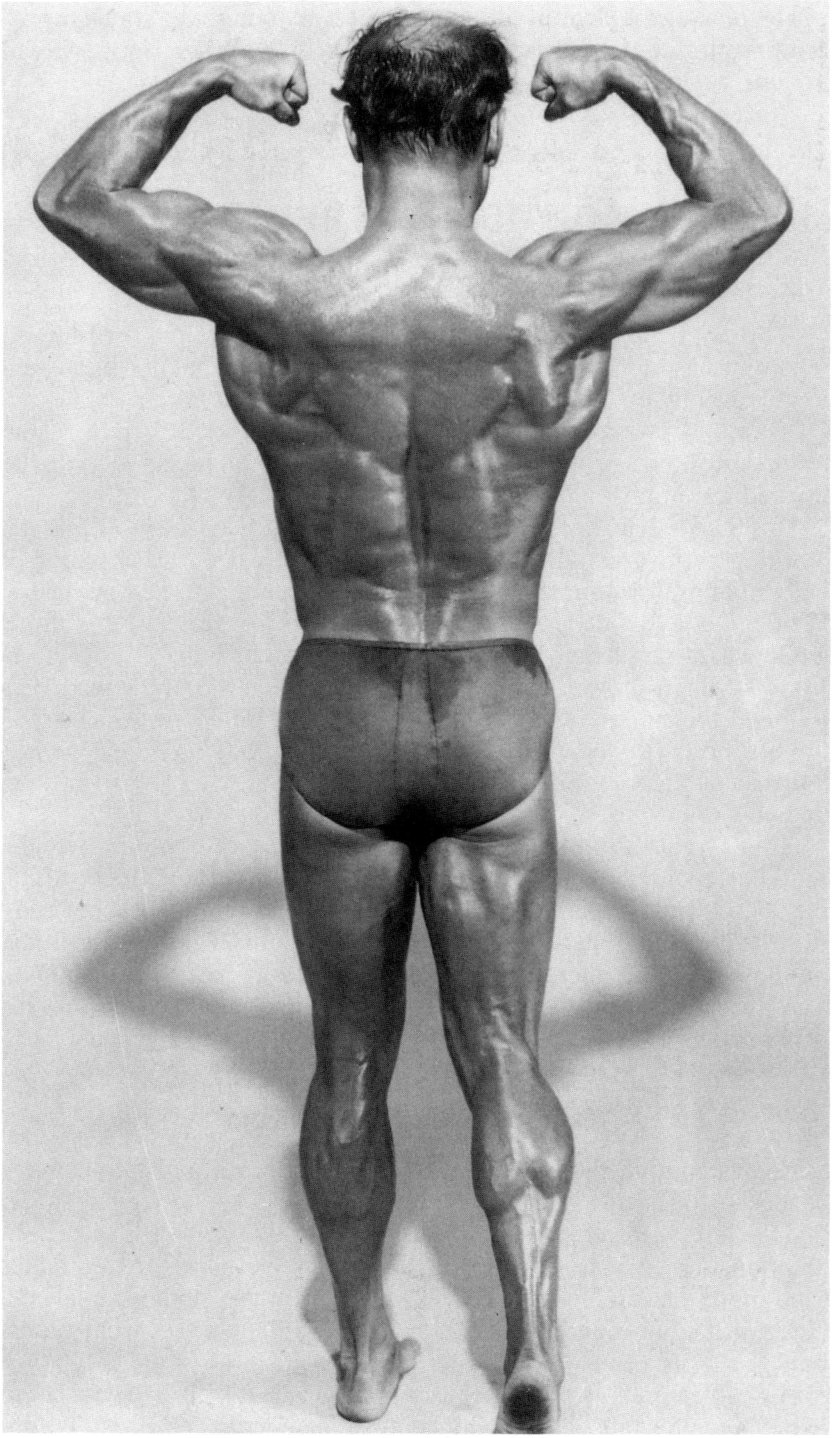

Another photo backstage at the 1978 Past-40 Mr. America. *Photo by Dave Sauer.*

bananas, carrots and bread; he drinks nothing but water. That may sound boring, but I believe him when he says he enjoys every meal. As readers know, I eat basically the same meals each day as well.

Obviously, my Swedish friend, through trial and error, has found a diet and exercise program that works for him. He's taken bits and pieces from Joe Weider, me, Arne Tammer and probably a lot of other people. He took what made sense to him and combined it to form his own unique system. It's his personal program and that, no doubt, is why it works so well — for him. He's undergone a psychological process of ownership. It's a process that often spells the difference between success and failure for those trying to become lean and fit.

The Ownership Principle

Most readers, I'm sure, have heard the dismal statistic that at least 95% of those who manage to lose weight gain it all back — and then some. That number is skewed. "The statistics we have come from clinical settings where you get the people with the toughest problems," says Kelly Brownell, Ph.D., codirector of the Obesity Research Clinic at the University of Pennsylvania. Nevertheless, it's common knowledge that most people fail to maintain their weight loss. Some do succeed, however. *Tufts University Diet & Nutrition Letter* told recently of a common link in the success stories. You guessed it: the ownership principle.

That's what Dr. Susan Olson, director of psychological services at the Southwest Bariatric Nutrition Center in Scottsdale, Arizona, and Dr. Robert Colvin of the Southern Illinois University School of Medicine found when they studied 54 adults who had lost at least 20% of their bodyweight and maintained their losses for a minimum of two years.

Olson and Colvin found plenty of variation in why and how these people succeeded. But there was one common denominator: They each found their own method for shedding pounds and keeping them off, a method with which they were comfortable, and which worked for them. Like my Swedish friend, they didn't rely on someone else's program. They developed their own.

That may sound too simple, but Olson said that many dieters find it much more comfortable to rely on external controls, such as weight-loss programs that dictate how to act. That mind-set allows the potential weight loser to feel that it's not really "up to him," that "cheating" reflects upon someone other than himself, that the control, the rules, the entire process are all out of his hands. Besides being untrue, such thoughts undermine a person's confidence in the weight loss solution. As the old adage says, "a person convinced against his will is of the same opinion still." That means, of course, that the dieter soon goes back to his old fattening ways.

"It's a matter of what people are really willing and not willing to do," Olson explains. My Swedish correspondent is not willing to lift weights for sets and reps; but calisthenics, running on the track in all manner of attire — rain or shine — and a low-fat diet suit him just fine. That's why the routine works for him. He made the rules, and he alone is responsible for the results. It's his program. He owns it.

"In short," the editors of *Diet & Nutrition Letter* concluded, "it's not the technique you choose to lose weight but how you view it."

DON'T GAMBLE WITH YOUR GUT

Stack the deck in your favor by dealing healthy foods

Q: *I've been overweight most of my life. The times when I've maintained optimal bodyweight have been few and far between. With the help of bodybuilding, I went from 145 as a freshman in high school to 185 rather bulky pounds at graduation. During six years of college my weight was as low as 165 (with the help of "speed") and as high as 213 after a bout of binge eating. Now, at age 27, I've kick boxed, jogged and dieted down to my present weight of 179. I'm 5 feet 11 and have a mesomorphic shape.*

Sadly, I still binge, miss workouts and generally sit on the sidelines in envy of athletes who have beaten the belly. I feel like I am losing ground, and I'm tired of living in fear of eating or missing a day of exercise.

I've resolved to redouble my efforts. My goal is to complete a marathon within the next year. To help me in that effort, I'd like to reduce my bodyweight to as low as 150. Can you help me?

A: It sounds like you are trying too hard. You seem to be at war with your diet and exercise regimen. I suggest a truce. Like many others, you are fighting nature rather than letting it work for you.

You sound like a victim of the "failure syndrome" that the authors of *Straight Talk About Weight Control* (Consumer Reports Books, 1991) describe as follows: "the familiar cycle of unrealistic vows to restrict food intake, eventual failure to adhere to the restrictions, and then giving up and overeating, feeling guilty and hopeless about ever achieving weight control." Failure, of course, is demoralizing. It destroys your enthusiasm for the challenge of lasting weight control. Considering your height and mesomorphic frame, your vow to lose another 30 pounds, down to 150, so you can post a good time in the marathon is probably unrealistic — a prescription for more failure and depression.

Appetite Control Mechanism

Let nature help you lose

Instead, stack the cards in your favor. Start by thinking in terms of eating a healthy diet rather than being *on a diet.* If you eat low-fat, high-fiber foods and avoid triggers or cues that cause you to eat unwisely, your natural appetite mechanism will regulate your calorie intake. You won't even know you are on a diet. Best of all, you'll gradually achieve optimal bodyweight automatically, without even trying.

As *Straight Talk About Weight Control* explains, one way the body regulates calorie intake is through a response linked to the feeling of an empty (or full) stomach and the appeal of food. Good smells and tastes or the sight of food sets off reflexes in the brain that make us want to eat. An empty stomach and intestines send hormonal and nervous signals to an important part of the brain called the hypothalamus. These messages that the stomach is empty and that good food is available trigger feeding behavior. Likewise, the hypothalamus registers when the stomach is full and sends the message that it is time to stop eating.

We don't know exactly how this feedback mechanism works in humans, but animal studies provide convincing evidence that it exists. Animals that have been overfed through a tube inserted into the stomach voluntarily decrease their food intake. What's more, blood serum extracted from such overfed animals, when injected into hungry animals, will decrease food intake. The blood evidently carries a message that it's time to stop eating.

You can make this mechanism work for you by eating foods with plenty of bulk but not many calories, such as vegetables, fruits and grains. You simply won't want to consume more calories than you need, especially if you eliminate things that encourage you to overeat. For example, don't leave extra food out where you can see it and be tempted. Cover up food in the refrigerator for the same reason. It also helps to eat slowly so your hypothalamus has time to do its job.

That doesn't mean never having an ice cream sundae or a candy bar. In fact, it's important to give yourself permission to stray occasionally. Go ahead and have some pizza if you really want it — and don't feel guilty. How fat you are is governed by what you usually eat, not by an occasional slip. In fact, I recommend that you eat fattening foods from time to time. It cuts down cravings and helps you eat healthy, low-calorie foods most of the time.

As for that marathon, you might be wiser to train for a shorter race. You'll probably enjoy a 5K or 10K competition more. Remember, the key is to set yourself up for success. It's much better to have a good experience in a shorter race than to disappoint yourself by dropping out of a marathon.

Inefficient Execise

An easy way to burn calories

Rather than drive yourself to run more miles in preparation for a marathon, I suggest you burn extra calories by becoming "inefficient" in your daily routine. Walk up the stairs instead of taking the elevator. Park across the parking lot at the supermarket. Stand when you can sit and sit when you could be lying down. For example, in airports when everyone else is sitting down, I make it a point to get up and walk around. Take it from me, over time these things make a difference — and they're easy.

Finally, don't overlook the role of weight training in keeping you lean. Resistance exercise doesn't burn as many calories as aerobic exercise, but it does maintain and build muscle mass. That's important because muscles burn calories and increase your metabolism. Muscle tissue burns calories even when you sleep.

You'll find many more details on staying lean without really trying — no calorie counting, no deprivation, no starvation, no dieting — in my latest book, *Lean For Life*. Take my advice and you'll never have to apologize to yourself again.

CHAPTER FIVE

WEIGHT TRAINING

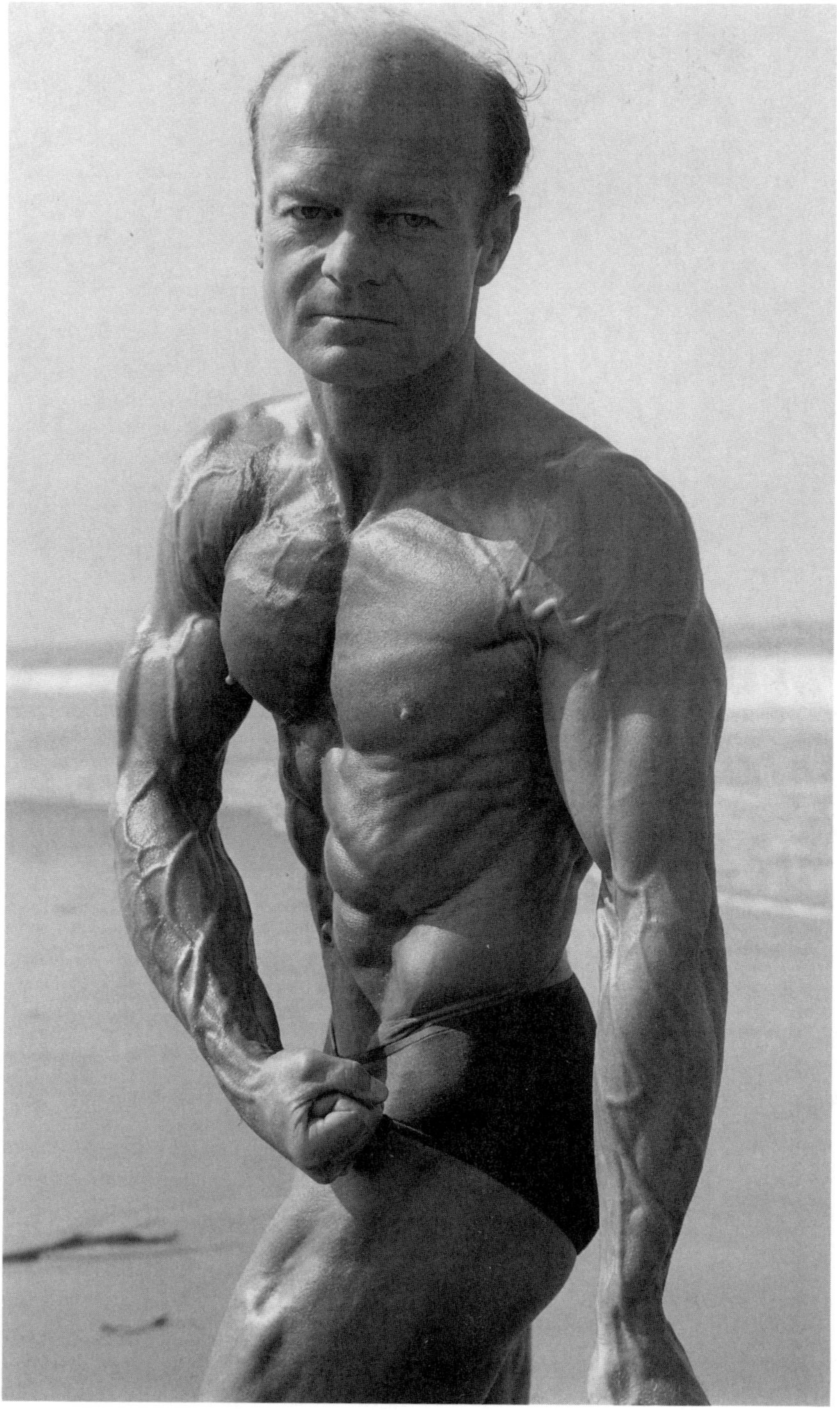

A few days after winning the Most Muscular Man, Best Abs and Best Legs at the 1979 Past-40 Mr. U.S.A. *Photo by Bill Reynolds.*

WEIGHT TRAINING 5

THE GROWING EDGE

Pump iron for physical and emotional growth

Q: *I'm all the things I shouldn't be. I really need direction about diet and exercise, so send me all five of your books. I need a drastic change in my life, and I need it yesterday!*

A: The books are on the way. They'll give you guidance on diet and exercise. Moreover, you may receive an exciting and, judging from the tone of your letter, urgently needed bonus.

I've often said that lifting weights is one of the most positive things I've ever done for myself. Weights helped me develop physically, but the benefits extend far beyond that. My years of training have helped me mentally and emotionally as well. As you'll discover from reading my books, lifting weights has helped me learn about myself and grow as a person.

You'll be interested to know that that's the basic theme of a new book on the psychology of lifting weights by Edward W.L. Smith, Ph.D.: *Not Just Pumping Iron* (Charles C. Thomas, 1989). Says Smith, a clinical psychologist with calluses on his hands to prove his long and intimate involvement with the barbell, "The greatest potential from lifting weights lies in doing so as a path for personal growth." Smith sees weight training as a microcosm for exploring concepts that hold true both in and out of the gym.

After you have a few months of weight training under your belt, you'll want to read *Not Just Pumping Iron.* It's filled with wonderful insights. You'll benefit now, however, from one of the concepts in the book. It's critical to growth in any area, but especially in bodybuilding, and it's often overlooked in training articles. Let me tell you about the "growing edge."

Grow With Overload

In any process we think in terms of the next step, the step beyond where we have been. This is the growing edge, the limit we are working to extend. In bodybuilding the growing edge is the boundary between what you have attained physically and what you are training to achieve. The growing edge is the boundary between your personal best in the bench press and the new record you're shooting for, or the boundary between your 15-inch arms and the 16-inch guns you're working to achieve.

Most beginning bodybuilders start training as hard as they can every workout. This works fine — at first. Then comes the sticking point. That's when you need to know about the growing edge. Bodybuilding progress, like progress in any other activity, is irregular; it's full of peaks, valleys and plateaus. Let's explore the ebb and flow of the growing edge in weight training.

The first thing to know is that growth occurs by extending the edge gradually. In bodybuilding, growth comes in small steps. We grow by gradually adding weight to our lifts. This is the Overload Training Principle. The body overcompensates for a particular lifting stress by muscular growth. So, rather than simply becoming accustomed to a particular poundage, the body grows from that lift to the point of being able to do that poundage plus a little more. You grow by increasing your poundage gradually, in small increments.

Don't Overtrain

Secondly, to gain muscular size and strength, you must lift progressively heavier weights. In the words of Smith, "Working too far behind the growing edge results in a lack of growth." In short, to grow you must overload your muscles. If you can squat 10 times with 200 pounds, you won't improve by doing 10 reps with 150. To grow you must extend yourself periodically by adding weight or repetitions; you have to do 200 pounds 11 times or increase the weight to 205.

Note, I said you must extend yourself "periodically." Listen to Dr. Smith again: "Too much time spent at one's growing edge without respite, results in arrest of progress and a feeling of growing stale." You must allow yourself to recover both physically and psychologically. If you max out too often, your progress will stall. It varies from person to person, but most people gain best by training a lift heavy once a week, and then a second or third time each week, but with less intensity. This is the hard-day, easy-day system you'll read about in *Ripped 2.*

The next principle is implicit in what I've already said, but it's important enough to focus on separately. Forcing too far beyond the growing edge, increasing your poundages too much, usually results in a loss of previous growth, or as Dr. Smith puts it, a "backlash." If your best in a lift is 100 pounds, it won't pay you to jump to 125. That's too much; you'll fail. You won't progress, and you may lose ground or injure yourself. The growing edge can't be forced; it must be coaxed forward, gradually, in small increments.

Two Steps Forward, One Back

Finally, don't expect to make continuous progress. A lifter must push for a while, back off, and then push again. Sticking points and setbacks are inevitable. Progress at the growing edge is not linear. As Dr. Smith says: "The growing edge evolves by going two steps forward, one back."

That's why, in *Ripped 3,* I suggest training in four-week phases or periods. You gradually increase your poundages every week for about a month, then you back off, lower the weights, and push forward again. Basically, that's what periodization is about.

There you have it. That's the growing edge phenomenon. Understand the nature of the growing edge, and you'll be well on your way to success in bodybuilding. My guess is that you'll also be on the path to personal growth.

MUSCLE AEROBICS

Aerobic benefits without muscle loss

Q: *I have two related questions: 1) Why couldn't one do a power/ mass program for the upper extremities and an endurance-based program for the lower? There seems to be a question whether making gains in both is feasible. 2) Dr. Fred Hatfield's book* Power *clearly states that weightlifters working for size and strength should not engage in aerobic exercise. This is contrary to the recommendation of many bodybuilders. What is your view?*

A: Have you ever seen anyone with an upper body like Lee Haney's and a lower body like Olympic and Boston Marathon winner Gelindo Bordin's? I haven't. I think such a physique would look strange, and I doubt that such a combination exists or is even possible. The body functions as a unit, responding best to a unified exercise program. You can't sleep for only half of your body and, likewise, I don't believe you could successfully train your upper body for size and strength and your lower body for endurance.

Your body mirrors your lifestyle. If you train like a marathon runner, you'll probably end up looking like one — with strong legs and a relatively undeveloped upper body, without much muscle mass — development suitable for running 26-plus miles. On the other hand, if you train like a weightlifter, you'll probably end up with big muscles and the appropriate mass suited for lifting heavy weights.

In these two extremes, the body receives a clear signal one way or the other: to adjust for endurance or for strength. The problem comes when the body gets competing, possibly mutually exclusive, messages;

it doesn't know whether to adapt for endurance (slow-twitch fibers and small muscles) or strength (fast-twitch fibers and large muscles). So it does neither very well.

That's why Fred Hatfield is probably correct in thinking that aspiring world-champion powerlifters should not do aerobic exercise. Bodybuilders, however, are required to be leaner than powerlifters. And, as I explain at length in *Ripped 2* and *Ripped 3,* bodybuilders need the aid of aerobic exercise to achieve maximum leanness. Plus, total fitness, with optimum strength *and* endurance, requires both weight training and aerobics. The trick is combining the two without sending mixed messages to the muscles.

All Or None

Muscle fibers operate on an all-or-none principle, which works hand in hand with the use-it-or-lose-it principle. My dentist has a sign on the wall that says, "Floss only the teeth you plan to keep." It's the same with muscle. If you don't use them, you'll lose them. (That's particularly true when you are dieting to lose fat. If you're not careful more than 50% of your loss will be lean tissue — muscle. The way to maximize fat loss and prevent loss of muscle is to train with weights.)

Muscles are made up of fibers that contract. When an individual muscle fiber is stimulated by a nerve impulse, it contracts completely or not at all. A muscle fiber is either completely "on" or completely "off." There's no such thing as a partial contraction of an individual fiber. Muscle fibers work as hard as possible — or not at all.

Why then can we contract the muscle at different intensities? Not because fibers are contracting at the different intensities (as we said, individual muscle fibers don't function that way), but because the brain calls only on the number of muscle fibers it needs for a given task. Those muscle fibers contract with all their might, and the remaining muscle fibers do nothing at all. Muscle fibers that aren't used remain small and weak. If you've ever had an arm or leg in a cast, you know how muscles atrophy from lack of use.

Even if you're active, some muscle fibers may never be called upon, so will never grow larger and stronger. What's the best way to contract your muscle fibers, all of them? Weight train, of course. No other form of exercise allows you to systematically exercise and develop so many muscles, and thus so many muscle fibers, in the body. Nothing else comes even close. No fitness program is complete unless it includes weight training for the whole body. To paraphrase my dentist, weight train only the muscles you plan to keep. (See *Ripped 2* for details on how to put the all-or-none law to work in your weight training program.)

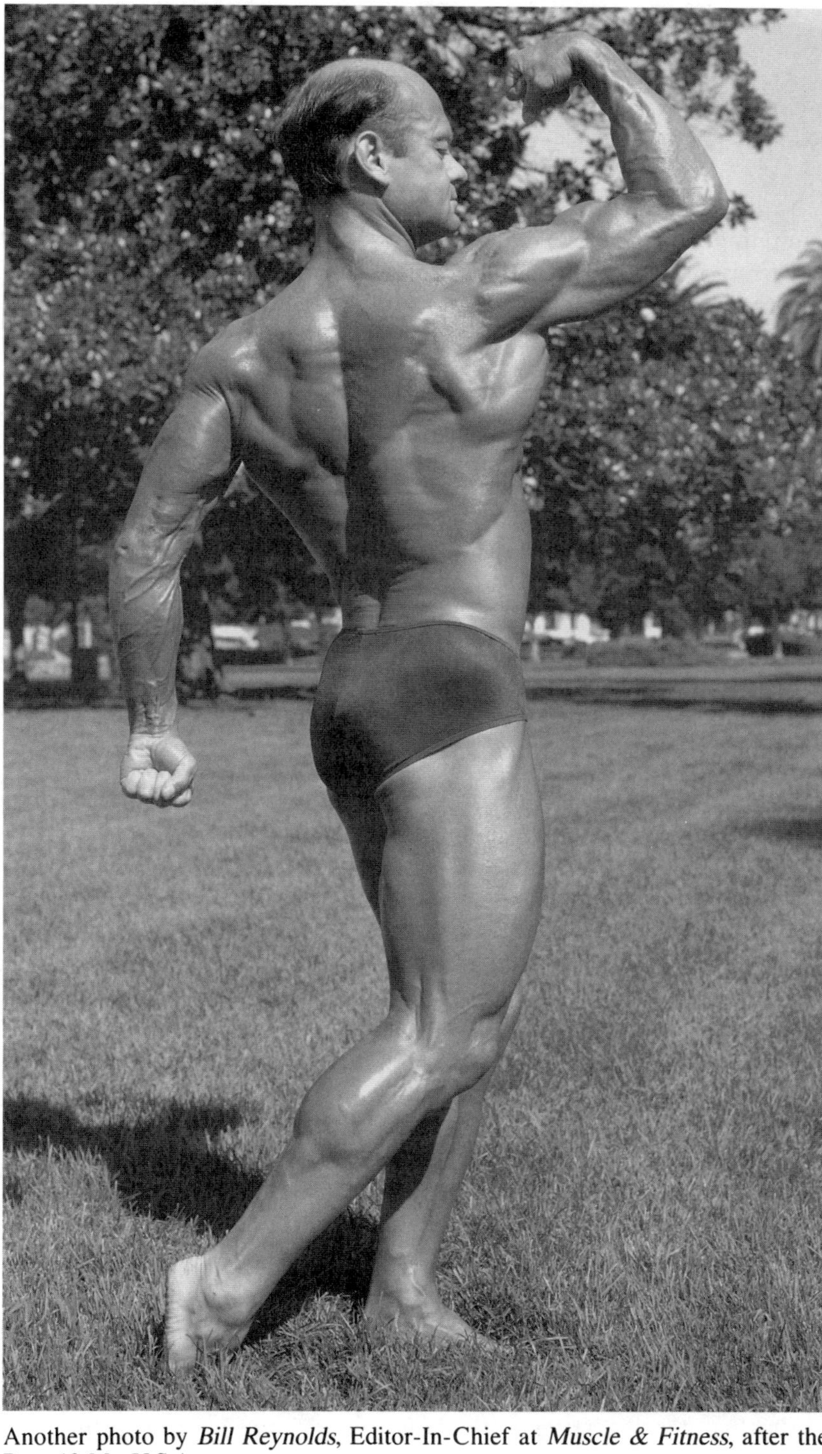

Another photo by *Bill Reynolds*, Editor-In-Chief at *Muscle & Fitness*, after the Past-40 Mr. U.S.A.

Aerobic Guidelines

As for the other important component of fitness, aerobic conditioning, here are my guidelines for bodybuilders. They're designed to give you the benefits of aerobic exercise without retarding your muscle gains.

1) Limit strenuous aerobic exercise to 30 minutes per session, excluding warm-up and cool-down, 3-4 times a week. This rule keeps you from overdosing on aerobics to the detriment of your bodybuilding program. Prolonged endurance exercise can destroy muscle tissue. Keep aerobic sessions short and this won't happen.

2) Practice different forms of aerobic exercise to distribute the stress to different parts of the body. This also prevents overtraining on aerobics. Train your whole body, arms and legs, using different forms of aerobic exercise (running, biking, rowing, climbing, skiing, etc.). Variety allows the exercised muscles to recover and keeps aerobic exercise from wearing down any one bodypart.

3) Include bursts of high-intensity muscular effort in every aerobic session. This involves your fast-twitch muscle fibers. They're the ones that hypertrophy even when you're doing aerobics. For example, when you run or bike, include some sprinting in your program. This reminds the muscles that you're a bodybuilder — not a marathoner — and you need and want to keep the muscles that were produced by weight training. The idea is to use your muscles so you won't lose them.

This is what I call "muscle aerobics." It's the way a bodybuilder can derive the fat-burning benefits of aerobic exercise, but avoid the muscle-wasting drawbacks. (For more details on muscle aerobics, including specific routines, please refer to *Ripped 3*.)

NEVER TOO OLD

Weight training keeps you young

Q: *I'm 47. Back in my 30s, I ran seriously until I burned out. After listening to my wife and others say I looked like a refugee from a concentration camp, I stopped exercising altogether.*

In my early 40s I began training again, this time lifting weights but running less. I've gained 10 pounds of lean muscle mass. I'm quite fit and lean but still a little on the light side (160 pounds at 6 feet).

The fitness director at the YMCA encourages me to keep lifting; she says I'll continue to gain muscle over time — and that strength training becomes increasingly important as I get older.

But I've heard that it's impossible to build muscle mass at my age. Am I getting too old to benefit from weight training?

A: Let's hear it for your fitness instructor! She obviously keeps up with the latest research. For years, the research community focused on endurance training. Exercise was practically a synonym for aerobic activities. The benefits of weight training were looked on as largely cosmetic.

Well, things have changed — and how! Landmark studies at the USDA Human Nutrition Research Center on Aging at Tufts University showed that people past middle age are able to gain muscle and increase strength by as much as 200%. What's more, muscle and strength, the elements most directly affected by weight training, are the key controllable physiological factors associated with aging.

This dramatic new evidence on the benefits of strength training is collected in the new book *Biomarkers* by William J. Evans, Ph.D., and Irwin H. Rosenberg, M.D., professors of nutrition and medicine at Tufts. (Simon & Schuster, 1991).

Biomarkers

To paraphrase Satchel Paige, the ageless baseball pitcher, biomarkers are those things that tell how old you would be "if you didn't know how old you was." Evans and Rosenberg isolated 10 of those signposts of vitality that can be altered for the better by changes in a person's lifestyle. Here they are:

1) Muscle mass
2) Strength
3) Basal metabolic rate
4) Bodyfat percentage
5) Aerobic capacity
6) Blood-sugar tolerance
7) Cholesterol/HDL ratio
8) Blood pressure
9) Bone density
10) Ability to regulate internal temperature

Surprise, surprise — at least in some people — all 10 biomarkers can be revived or improved through weight training.

To help people understand how strength training affects the biomarkers, Evans and Rosenberg coined the term "sarcopenia" to describe an ailment that afflicts many old people and deprives them of their independence. "Sarco" refers to flesh, "penia" means a reduction in amount. So sarcopenia describes an overall weakening of the body caused by a change in body composition in favor of fat and at the expense of muscle.

That's just the opposite of what bodybuilders seek — which is maximum muscle with minimum fat. That's what sarcopenia sufferers lack. Their bodies have wasted away over the years through a lack of activity. What's the cure? You got it: strength training.

Muscle Mass

Evans and Rosenberg say that the first biomarker, muscle mass, is responsible for the vitality of your whole physiological apparatus. Muscle mass and strength, the second signpost, are our primary biomarkers. They're the lead dominoes, so to speak. When they start to topple, the other biomarkers soon follow. On the other hand, when muscle mass and strength are maintained, the other indicia are likewise maintained. That's where strength training comes to our aid. Aerobic exercise and diet are important, but strength training, according to Evans and Rosenberg, is pivotal if you want to stay young longer.

The average person's lean body mass declines with age, with the rate of loss usually accelerating around age 45. It doesn't have to be that way, however. the main factor responsible for how much muscle and strength we have is how much we use our muscles. That's old news to bodybuilders.

Strength Training

What is new is research showing that old people can still increase strength and muscle mass; they respond to strength training the same as a young person. This new research allows Evans and Rosenberg to state boldly: "A decline in muscle strength and size is not inevitable."

Conventional thinking has been that age somehow decreases the ability of the muscles to get bigger in response to strength training. Not so, say these researchers.

They had 12 older men, ages 60-72, train with weights at 80% of their one repetition maximum for three days a week for 12 weeks. The amount of weight lifted was increased every week, providing progressive overload.

The results? Quadriceps strength more than doubled, and hamstring strength tripled. Computed tomography and muscle biopsy showed a remarkable 12% collective increase in muscle size. "The amount of hypertrophy was as much as we would expect to see in young people doing the same amount of exercise," the writers observed.

In another study 10 men and women, ages 87-96, trained at 80% of their one rep maximum for eight weeks. Their results, according to Evans and Rosenberg, were even more startling. The subjects' muscle strength almost tripled and the size of their thigh muscles grew by more than 10%.

That is amazing when you consider that these were frail, institutionalized, elderly people. One 93-year-old study participant observed: "I feel as though I were 50 again... Pills won't do for you what exercise does!"

Still think you may be too old to build muscle mass at the age of 47?

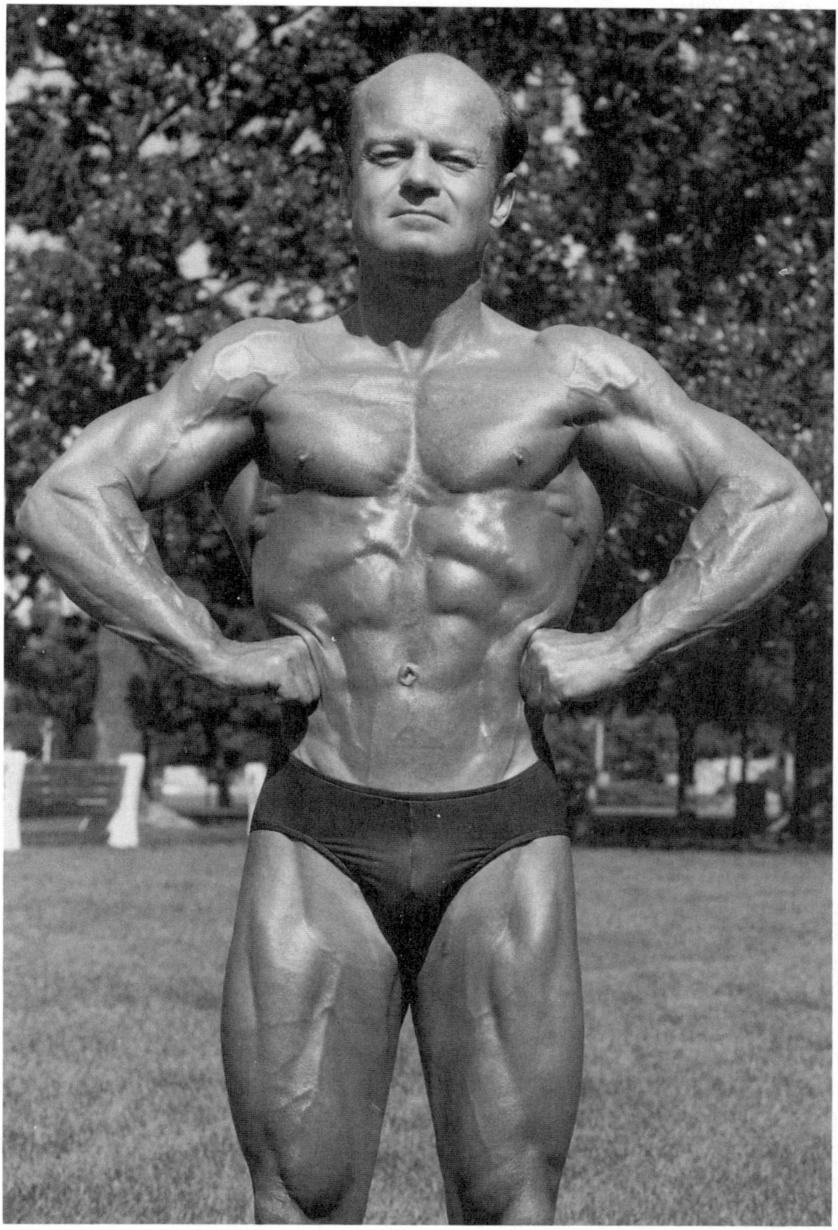

Photo by Bill Reynolds.

RX FOR HEALTH: BODYBUILDING

Physicians now know total fitness is more than aerobics

Did you notice? During the 1980s, the way the medical community viewed strength training/bodybuilding changed dramatically. Up to that time, the doctors' prescription for fitness was short and simple: aerobic exercise. Jog, bike or swim — that was about it. Then things began to change. Slowly but surely, weight training worked its way up the medical-advice list and, finally, took its place on the doctor's prescription pad as an equal partner with aerobic exercise.

In short, we have witnessed the birth of a new concept in exercise: "balanced fitness." In April 1990, the influential American College of Sports Medicine altered its exercise guidelines for the first time in 12 years, recommending a "well-rounded" program that includes strength training along with aerobic exercise.

My first inkling that a change was afoot came in the form of a call from a Pennsylvania orthopedic surgeon, shortly after the publication of *Ripped 2*, my second book, in which I explained that a combination of weight training and aerobic exercise is the best way to achieve permanent leanness. The doctor reported that following my advice he had lost 30 pounds. He felt like a new man. The change in his lifestyle, he predicted, was going to add years to his lifespan. He said something I'll always remember: "I never thought a doctor, like myself, could learn so much about his body from an attorney!" The next major hint that bodybuilding was gaining in status with the medical profession came a few years later when Dr. Arno (Arnie) Jensen called from the Cooper Clinic to invite me to come to Dallas for a complete health and fitness evaluation. Arnie said that my ideas on diet and exercise, as expressed in *Muscle & Fitness* and my books, were much the same as his. Significantly, he told me that the Cooper Clinic gym now had a fully equipped weight training area. He also said I would be the first high-level bodybuilder to be tested at the clinic.

Call From Mecca

As many of you know, Dr. Kenneth Cooper, the founder of the Cooper Clinic, wrote the book *Aerobics*, which was published in 1968 and was largely responsible for the joggers that flooded the streets across the country and around the world during the '70s and '80s. So you can see that a call to a bodybuilder from the birthplace of the aerobics movement was a real breakthrough.

My test at the Cooper Clinic confirmed Jensen's belief that a combination of weight training and aerobics, balanced training, would produce very positive results. For example, my performance on the treadmill put me 2½ minutes above the 99th percentile for men 50-59 and in the top group for men of any age. Jensen pronounced my overall health "superb."

In 1990 the Institute for Aerobics Research, an offshoot of the Cooper Clinic, published *The Strength Connection,* a book about balanced fitness. Cooper wrote in the foreword: "At the Institute for Aerobics Research we're learning more every day about the importance of strong muscles and bones. The purpose of this book is to emphasize the benefits of balanced fitness: regular physical activity that includes strength training... in addition to aerobic conditioning.

Superhealth 2000

The latest confirmation that the doctors favored balanced fitness came a few months ago when I received a call from Dharma Singh Khalsa, MD, of the Maricopa Medical Center in Scottsdale, Arizona. Khalsa asked me to make a presentation on my approach to fitness at a conference to be sponsored by his group, the department of medical education, and the University of Arizona College of Medicine. Khalsa's workshop, the one in which I was being asked to participate, was entitled "Superhealth 2000: The Amazing New Technology of Living Long and Well." Wow! They were asking a bodybuilding lawyer to talk to medical doctors about superhealth! Needless to say, I accepted.

In Scottsdale, I told them that the benefits of muscle development go beyond having more strength and an attractive body. I said that a combination of weight training and aerobic exercise is the best way to lose bodyfat and keep it off. Strength training, I explained, plays an important role in fat control because increasing the amount of muscle in the body causes an increase in the basal metabolic rate and an associated increase in calorie expenditure. I said total fitness comes only from balanced training, aerobic exercise combined with weight training.

Additional Benefits

And here are some additional benefits of strength training that captured the interest of the doctors:

- Strength training can have beneficial effects on blood cholesterol levels. Research by Dr. Linn Goldberg at the University of Oregon showed that strength training elevated HDL (the good cholesterol) levels and decreased LDL (the bad cholesterol) in previously sedentary men and women.
- Strength training builds strong bones. That's because bones, like muscles, respond to the overload principle — they get stronger and thicker the more they are used or exercised. Obviously, this had important implications for women who have a high risk of developing osteoporosis.

• Strength training improves the quality of life. Most people start losing muscle tissue (and gaining bodyfat) in their 30s. Weight training can reverse this trend. Maintaining muscle strength, in addition to improving athletic performance, makes everyday activities easier.

• Strength training enhances self-esteem. The psychological benefits can be one of the biggest incentives to following a balanced exercise program. Developing a stronger, leaner, more attractive body makes you feel good about yourself.

So congratulations, *M&F* readers, you're in the forefront of the fitness trend of the '90s: balanced fitness.

RETURN ON INVESTMENT

Or how to get results in less time

Q: *I have trouble accepting what I read in your new book,* Lean For Life. *You recommend only four hours of training a week. What's more, you advocate only one hard set of each exercise after warm-up. I'm sorry, but that doesn't sound like enough training to produce results. How do you justify such a small amount of training? Have you given up your quest for ultimate fitness?*

A: Absolutely not. As a lawyer with many other interests and responsibilities, I've always sought maximum results with a minimum expenditure of time. I understand your skepticism, however. You are accustomed to hearing about champion bodybuilders who train practically every day, often splitting their workouts into morning and evening sessions. These people no doubt train many more hours each week than I recommend. Terry Todd, the extremely knowledgeable co-editor of *Iron Game History* published at the University of Texas at Austin, observed recently that many bodybuilders spend four or five times as many hours in the gym as I do. He's correct, of course. Doesn't that prove your point? No, I don't believe so.

George Sheehan, MD, the venerable old man of running, expressed the basic rationale for my recommendations in his new book, *George Sheehan on Running to Win* (Rodale Press, 1992). Sheehan says of elite runners who average well over 100 miles per week, "Such training programs do not make champions, they discover them."

100-Mile-A-Week Runners

"These people are animals!"

Speaking at a running clinic where he followed a panel of 100-mile-per-week runners, Sheehan took the microphone and said: "Forget everything these people told you. They're not like us. They're animals!"

Only gifted athletes can survive such training methods, Sheehan explained. Ordinary people, on the other hand, end up sick or injured.

Sheehan points out that Roger Bannister broke the four-minute-mile barrier on only five hours of training each week. Bannister later wrote that an additional 10 seconds of improvement would require four times as much training. In other words, you reach a point of diminishing returns. The greatest percentage of improvement comes from the first few hours of training each week. Training beyond that results in minimum change — and dramatically increases the likelihood of staleness or injury.

The same holds true for weight training. As you may know, Bulgaria has produced the world's best Olympic lifters in recent years on a regimen of six-times-a-day heavy training. This may work for genetically gifted, young athletes with unlimited time to train but, as I wrote in *Lean For Life,* "Most people, even if they had the time and inclination, would be destroyed — physically and mentally — by such training."

The Bulgarians are an extreme example, of course, but they illustrate that champions often emerge from training programs that would leave the average person a wreck. Most lifters would realize better gains from far less training. Moreover, shorter programs are more enjoyable, and allow time for a normal life outside the gym.

As you know, in *Lean For Life* I recommend that maximum-intensity workouts be limited to two a week. Any more than that will depress your immune system, according to Dr. David C. Neiman, associate professor of health, leisure and exercise science at Appalachian State University in North Carolina. Neiman's advice is based on a study of some 2,300 runners who entered the 1987 Los Angeles Marathon. In the two months before the race, 40% got sick. Those who ran more than 60 miles a week got sick twice as often, according to Neiman, as those who ran less than 20 miles a week. Plus, more than 13% of those who completed the marathon were sick within a week, compared to only 2% of those who trained for the event but didn't compete.

High Mileage

Killer-cell caution

Why did the high-mileage runners get sick more often? Neiman said it's because high mileage depresses the activity of the natural killer cells, the cells that kill foreign invaders in the body, such as viruses and bacteria. His work on a smaller group of runners showed that natural killer cell activities fell by more than 30% for almost six hours after a long, hard workout.

I've often gotten sick myself after prolonged periods of hard training. I've found that limiting hard training sessions to twice a week keeps

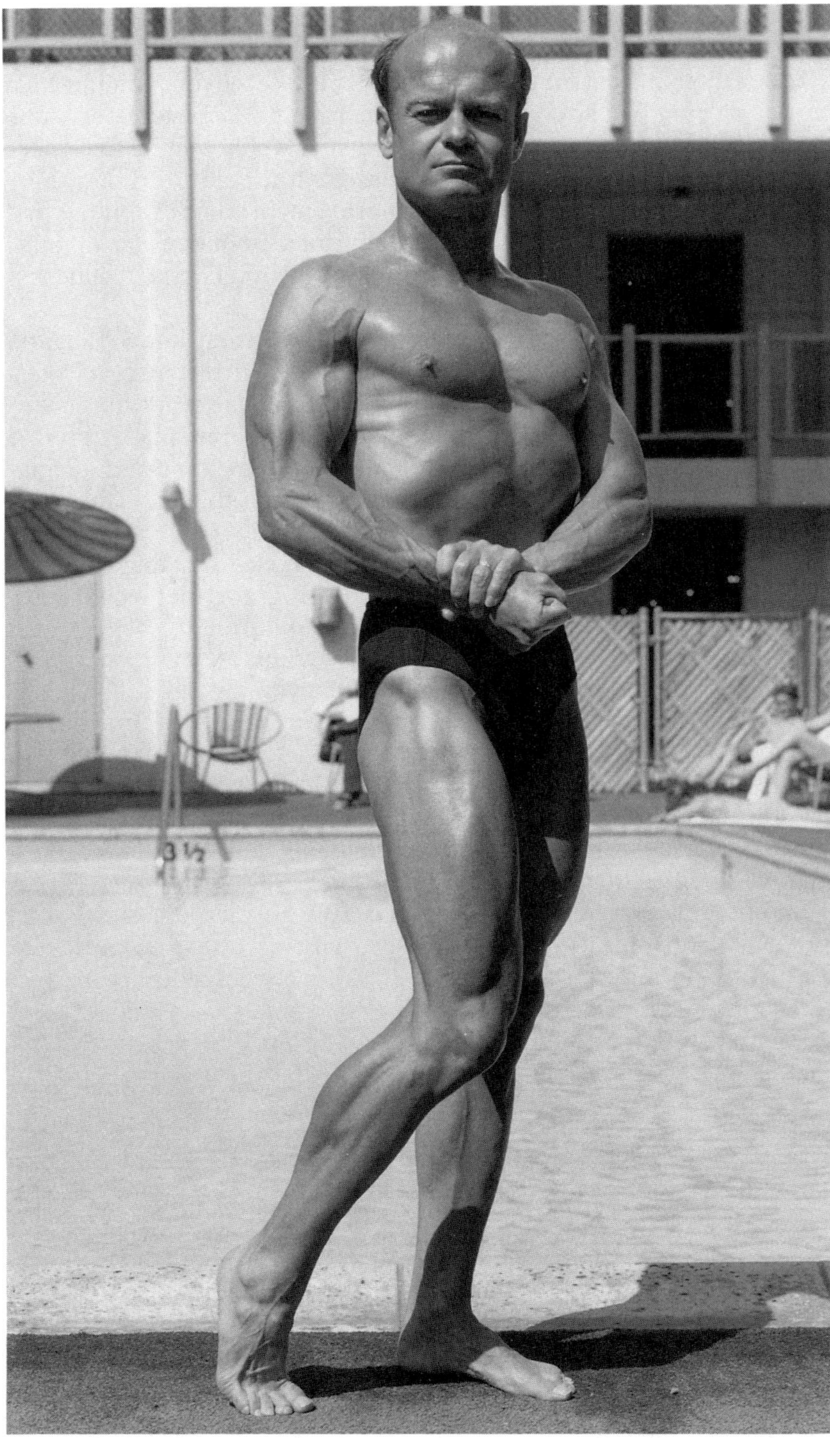

July 1977. *Photo by Dave Sauer.*

me well. So I think Neiman's advice is right on target.

Turning to your second point, let me tell you about a recent experience that convinced me — again — that best results come from doing only one hard set of each exercise after warm-up.

I've never been one to do very many sets. I find it boring to do the same exercise over and over. Nevertheless, for a change, I was doing three hard sets per exercise in a recent workout cycle: 12 reps with a medium poundage, eight with a heavy weight and a final back-off set of 20 repetitions. I had been increasing the poundage on all three sets for several weeks. So I thought I was performing close to my limit on all three sets. Then, one day, I decided to do only the first set and forego the other two. The result was eye-opening.

After a few easy warm-up sets, I loaded the bar with a weight I thought was my 12-rep maximum for this particular exercise, the deadlift. When I reached 12 reps I was still going strong, so I continued. I did 13, 14 and, finally, I ground out 15 reps!

Obviously, in my earlier workout, I was holding back on the 12-rep set. Whether I knew it or not, I was pacing myself. Subconsciously, I was saving my energy for the two sets to follow. However, when I cut back to one set, I focused totally on that set without thinking about the sets to follow. That freed me to make a better effort; it produced a more intense and, therefore, more productive set.

Many others have had similar experiences. For example, personal trainer Barry Rubin told me that his clients were getting such good results from my one-set method that he decided to try it himself. Barry reported: "I did 12 reps in the bench press with 250. My previous best was 225!"

Why not give my recommendations a try? You've got nothing to lose, except a lot of unproductive hours in the gym.

HARD TRAINING BLUES

Doing more can leave you with less

Q: *I'm a 21-year-old female and have been working out for two years. At first, like most beginners, I just wanted to tone up. Now, I'm interested in competitive bodybuilding.*

Presently, I'm working out three times a week for 60 to 90 minutes, but I'll shortly be increasing to four times a week. I always try to give maximum effort while being careful to use correct form. However, I often get impatient when I don't get fast results.

The problem is that after training my body is completely exhausted. I have no energy left to perform other tasks. All I want to do is sleep.

I get plenty of sleep at night and eat a balanced diet. Do you have any thoughts on why I'm always fatigued?

A: Your situation is not unusual. Enthusiastic bodybuilders, like you, frequently get carried away with their early success. They make great gains in the beginning — almost everybody does — and when the gains slow down — as usually happens — they, quite logically, think the answer is to train more. Unfortunately, that often makes things worse. Like you, they end up in a state of exhaustion, and with little else to show for the extra effort.

High Intensity Trap

Balance intensity against volume

Charlie Francis, the Canadian coach whose runners set 32 world records and won nine Olympic medals — Francis himself was the number five sprinter in the world in 1971 — says 90 percent of his time is spent holding athletes back to prevent overtraining and only 10 percent motivating them to do more work (*The Charlie Francis Training System*, TBLI Publications, 1992). Francis explains that on a given day there is only so much central nervous system energy to expend. "When it's drained, it's drained." Plus, training at maximum intensity all the time, as you are doing, compounds the problem. Listen carefully to coach Francis: "The athlete usually wants to build on a spectacular workout and train even harder." This can lead to overtraining and injury. Francis continues, "If the previous workout has been spectacular, I will pull back and force an easier workout as a matter of principle." In other words, Francis advocates following hard workouts with less intense training sessions.

Is the advice of a sprint coach, you may ask, relevant for bodybuilders? As their muscular physiques suggest, sprinters have much in common with bodybuilders. Coach Francis' athletes, male and female, train with heavy weights. Ben Johnson, the well-known sprinter who began training under Francis in his mid-teens, has done 10 repetitions in the bench press with 352 and sets of six repetitions with 600 in the one-half squat. And get this, Francis says his female sprinters, who include the likes of world and Canadian record holder Angella Issajenko, are 90-95 percent as strong, pound for pound, as his male sprinters in the lower body and generally 60-65 percent as strong in the upper body. For example, his female sprinters are capable of power cleaning their own bodyweight for 3-5 repetitions.

High intensity training, according to Francis, is what allowed his athletes to become world record holders. He adds, however, that intensity must be balanced against volume. "The highest possible movement speeds or the heaviest weights deplete the central nervous system energy pool most quickly." That's why he insists that his athletes take it easy after a hard training session. This allows time for recovery and prepares the body to perform at even higher levels. "Don't go for more when that can lead to ending up with less," says Francis.

Classic Symptons

Rest is cure for overtraining

The general malaise that you are experiencing is a classic symptom of overtraining. As Dr. George Sheehan explained in *Running To Win* (Rodale Press, 1992), overtraining follows a typical pattern. Acute fatigue after training, as you describe, is the first symptom. If the athlete rests, recovery is rapid. Continuing to train despite fatigue, says Sheehan, leads to exhaustion. "Unless training is suspended, exhaustion may persist for weeks or even months."

Once an athlete gets to that stage, as it appears you have, he or she needs a period of complete rest. You say all you want to do is sleep. Dr. Sheehan says that's what you should do. He recommends using the hour a day usually spent in training to take a nap. "Continuing to train will only prolong the time the athlete needs to rest."

So, I suggest that you spend a few days napping instead of training. When your urge to sleep passes, substitute a daily walk for your workout. Do that until your enthusiasm for training simply forces you back into the gym. In other words, take your time recovering. Dr. Sheehan says you may need to rest for up to six weeks.

Less Is More

Hard-easy training sequence

When you are fully recovered and return to the gym, go ahead and up your training to four times a week — but with an important change. Take a cue from Charlie Francis. Train hard two days and back off on the other training sessions each week. For example, you might want to follow the four-day, push-pull split routine described in my book *Ripped 3*. In this routine, the body is divided into pushing and pulling muscles. The pushing muscles — thighs, calves, chest, shoulders and triceps — are trained on one day, and the pulling muscles — lower back, leg biceps, upper back, biceps and abs — the next day. To complete the four-day training cycle, the pushing and pulling muscles are trained a second time each week, again on separate days, *but with less intensity.*

You'll find that this hard-day/easy-day sequence will produce better results than trying to train hard every workout. What's more, you'll have energy left for other things; you won't be tired all the time. (*Ripped 2* tells the story of my own conversion, kicking and screaming all the way, to hard-easy training.)

MY SECRET WEAPON

Low reps and heavy weights develop explosive power

I recently told a group of coaches how, in 1954, I used a "secret weapon" to out-jump everyone in a state high school fitness competition. Speaking at the Second Annual Strength Clinic held at New Mexico State University, I related that I began my athletic career by winning the State High School Pentathlon Championship, a five-event contest consisting of push-ups, chin-ups, jump reach, bar vault and 300-yard shuttle run. I explained to the coaches how weight training gave me a leg up on the other competitors. I had a special advantage in the vertical jump, a test of leg and hip power, because I was using an exercise untried by the other competitors. My secret weapon was the Barbell Squat.

Even though I was only a junior in high school, I had already been squatting for a number of years. I used heavy weights and low reps (2-5) in the Squat to help me in the Olympic lifts. Heavy Squats, combined with the Snatch and Clean & Jerk, gave me the explosive power in the thighs, hips and lower back to jump higher than the others. Today, because it places such great stress on the leaping muscles of the body, the Squat forms the core of the training program of most athletes. That wasn't true when I was in high school, however. In fact, the pentathlon coach discouraged me from weight training. I had to lift on my own, at home.

In later years, there have been many more demonstrations of the explosive power developed by training the leaping muscles with low reps and heavy weights. The most recent was by 6′3″, 365-pound, Olympic lifter Mark Henry. The 22-year-old Texan, currently this country's top superheavyweight lifter, can easily dunk a basketball. Astonishingly, this behemoth participated in a Footlocker Slamfest in Phoenix and won enough prize money to put him behind the wheel of a new Jeep Cherokee.

Develops Fast Fibers

But there's a problem

As a teenager I really didn't know how my secret weapon worked. I just knew that weight training gave me the edge. I now know that resistance training, as performed by weightlifters and other power athletes, develops the fast-twitch muscle fibers, which contract two to three times as fast as fibers classified as slow twitch. It is these fast twitch fibers that allow sprinters, jumpers, shot putters and the like to perform in such explosive fashion. That's why coaches, such as Canada's Charlie Francis, use heavy weights for low repetitions in a few key exercises (the Squat, Bench Press and Power Clean, for example) to develop power, or strength plus speed.

Coaches face a dilemma, however. The problem is that most sports require a combination of power and endurance. As I explained in *Lean For Life*, endurance exercise can reduce or blunt strength development. It seems that there exists a continuum of muscle fiber types ranging from the slowest to the fastest contracting, and that aerobic training can result in the formation of more slow-twitch fibers. Conversely, heavy weight training can bring about an increase in fast-twitch fibers.

Muscle fiber distribution is still thought to be governed largely by genetic factors, but there appear to be some fibers that can take on fast-twitch or slow-twitch characteristics depending on the type of training they undergo. Coaches and athletes in sports that require a combination of strength and endurance — that includes most sports — must strike a careful balance between the two types of training. It's also important to bodybuilders, because fast-twitch fibers increase in size (hypertrophy) much more than do slow-twitch fibers.

Nevertheless, most athletes, even those at the extremes, can benefit from both types of training. For example, Steve Spence, America's top marathoner, was recently pictured in *Runner's World* doing a heavy Barbell Squat. Rather than doing many repetitions with light weights, Spence performs fewer repetitions (8-10) with the heaviest weights he can lift. At the opposite pole, Dorian Yates did 30 minutes of aerobics twice a day prior to his victory in the 1992 Mr. Olympia. The relevant question for most people is not whether to combine strength and endurance training, but how best to do it.

Weapon Reactivated

Hands-on demo convinces me

As part of the strength training clinic referred to above, New Mexico State Strength Coach John Taylor presented a hands-on demonstration of lifting techniques. Among other things, he had one of his athletes demonstrate proper form in the Power Clean, where a barbell is pulled from the floor to the shoulders in one movement. As suggested earlier, the Power Clean is one of the exercises emphasized by Coach Charlie Francis. For example, Mark McKoy, a 170-lb. sprinter and hurdler trained by Francis, does five reps in the Power Clean with 225 and a single with 285.

After seeing Coach Taylor's athletes lift — and remembering the strength training techniques used by Charlie Francis — I decided to reactivate my secret weapon. I incorporated Power Cleans and Low-Rep Squats into my workouts. I almost always include Squats, so the only change there was to increase the weight and lower the reps to 5 and under, but I haven't done the Power Clean in the last few years. I found that I was strong off the ground, because the Deadlift is a regular part of my routine, but I was surprisingly weak in the second pull to the

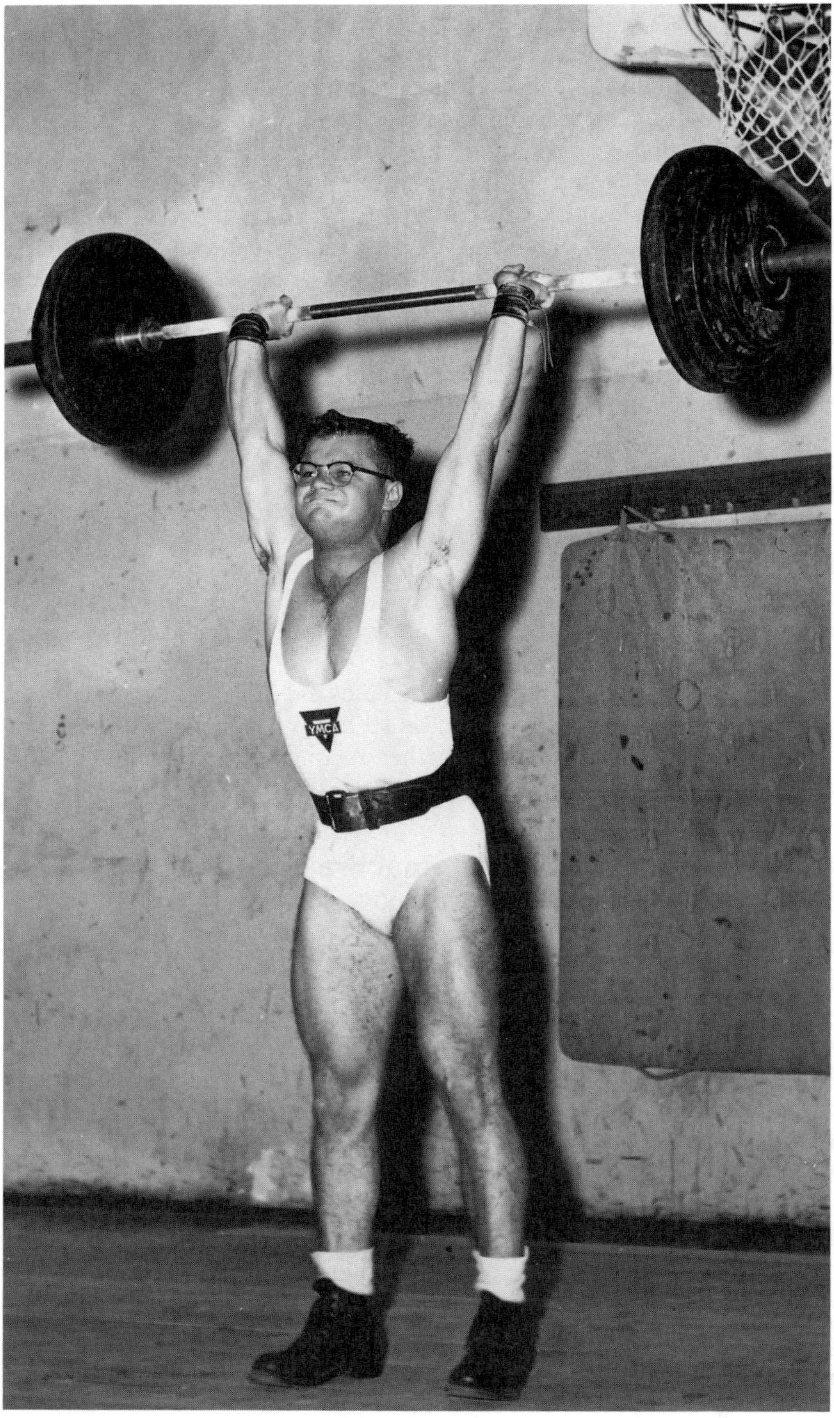

Doing the Clean & Jerk at one of my first Olympic lifting contests. This is the type of lifting that gave me the edge in high school sports.

shoulders. Happily, after a break-in period, my body has responded well to both exercises, and I am now making good progress. Plus, I'm having a good time. Squats are Squats, always hard, but it's really a joy to do a quick lift again. I can almost feel my intermediate fibers switching from slow to fast. It's great!

Why not try my secret weapon yourself? If you do, take a tip from Charlie Francis: Focus on quality, not volume. Two or 3 snappy low-rep sets, after warm up, are plenty. For instruction on proper performance of the Power Clean and other speed-strength building exercises, I recommend *Lift Your Way To Youthful Fitness* by Jan and Terry Todd (Little, Brown & Company, 1985). (*Lift* is available from Ripped Enterprises.)

CHAPTER SIX

AEROBICS

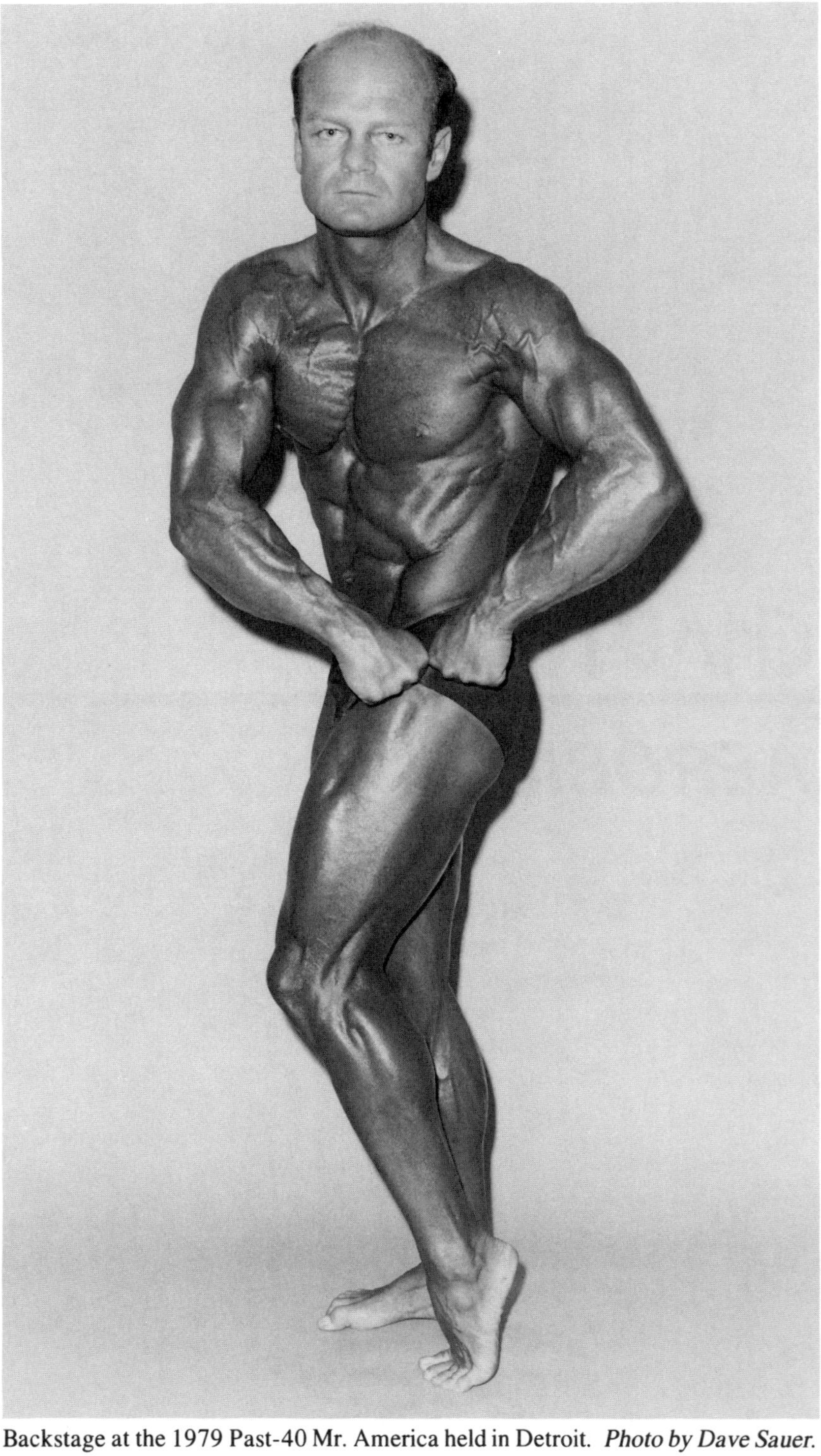

Backstage at the 1979 Past-40 Mr. America held in Detroit. *Photo by Dave Sauer.*

AEROBICS 6

FUN & FAT BURNING

Greater gains from interval training

Q: *For aerobic conditioning and fat loss, the strength and conditioning coach for a nearby pro hockey team suggests 5-10 minutes on each of various machines. I do this at my gym using the Air-Dyne, steps, bike, jogger and rower. This spreads the stress, as you recommend, and beats boredom. What do you think of this routine?*

A: I see both benefits and drawbacks. As you say, this workout spreads the stress to different parts of the body. That's good because it allows you to do more aerobic exercise and, therefore, burn more bodyfat without undue fatigue. It's also more enjoyable than doing the same thing continuously. The routine has a major flaw, however.

You must consider two important factors in formulating an aerobic exercise program. First, the training must be geared to overload the central circulatory system, primarily the heart and lungs. No doubt your program does that; I'm sure your heart rate and breathing are elevated continuously. Second, an effective program should place demands on the local circulation and "metabolic machinery" within specific muscles. In other words, you must challenge the aerobic mechanism within each individual muscle. This is where you may be falling short. By changing exercises every 5-10 minutes, you're probably not stimulating individual muscles sufficiently. The same muscles should be worked continuously for at least 15 minutes, and longer would be better.

The Specificity Principle

This is the specificity principle as applied to aerobic training. It explains why circuit weight training doesn't do a very good job of developing aerobic fitness; the aerobic mechanism within individual muscles is never really challenged. In short, to be good at a specific activity, you must practice that activity. Runners should run, rowers should row, skiers should ski.

To satisfy the need for specificity but still spread the stress and reduce boredom, I suggest that you stick to one machine each workout and do *intervals.* That's what I'm currently doing.

I do aerobics three times a week, rotating each workout between the Air-Dyne (a stationary bike with push-pull arm action), hiking or the treadmill, and the rower. It's not a good idea to rotate between more than three different aerobic exercises at any one time, however. With more exercises you experience a deconditioning effect before returning to the same exercise. Frequency — at least once a week on a particular exercise — is another requirement of effective conditioning.

Interval Training

Interval training is doing bursts of high-intensity activity — "repetitions" — separated by timed periods — "intervals" — of low-intensity recovery activity. Research has shown you can do more work this way than in a workout in which the exercise is performed at a steady pace. The reason is that the recovery intervals allow the removal of some lactic acid that accumulates in the muscles and makes them tired.

In one study, on one day researchers had their subject run at a speed that would normally exhaust him within five minutes. He covered 0.8 mile in four minutes during this continuous run and attained a maximal oxygen consumption of 5.6 liters per minute. The subject was exhausted at the end of the run; the lactic acid level in his blood was 150 milligrams per 100 milliliters.

On another day, the subject ran at the same speed, but for only 10 seconds at a time, followed by five-second "rest" intervals. With this protocol the subject ran for 30 minutes, including 20 minutes at the fast pace. He covered a total distance of four miles compared to less than five minutes and only 0.8 mile when the run was performed continuously! This is even more impressive when you consider that the average oxygen consumption throughout the 30-minute workout was 5.1 liters per minute compared to 5.6 during the continuous run. What's more, the lactic acid level remained low (44 versus 150 during the continuous run) even though the oxygen consumption remained quite high. In short, intervals allowed the subject to exercise five times longer than continuous running (20 minutes versus four) — at the same pace. Predictably, the fitness gains were also greater.

Two Studies

The *University of California, Berkeley Wellness Letter* (November 1988) gives the results of two studies that show the superior gains produced by interval training. At the University of Massachusetts Medical Center in Worchester, sedentary women rode stationary bicycles for 12 minutes three times a week. Half cycled at a constant speed and the others used computerized bikes that simulated progressively steeper hills (repetitions) and easy straightaways (intervals). The interval training procued an 11% increase in aerobic capacity, while the steady-pace rides produced only a 4% improvement. The *Wellness Letter* points out, however, that an 11% gain is far below the 18-25% you would expect from a conventional jogging regimen. "Moreover," they added, "the 12-minute sessions led to no change in bodyfat or weight." As the next study demonstrates, longer interval workouts are better.

Researchers at the University of Miami Human Performance Laboratory studied the results of aerobic dance sessions using interval training — 3-5 minutes of intense exercise alternating with three minutes of brisk walking or slow running — and steady-pace dance sessions. Both workouts lasted 35 minutes (not including warm-up and cool-down). Both groups exercised three times a week for 12 weeks. Interval training produced gains of 18% in aerobic capacity while the continuous sessions produced gains of only 8%. Unlike subjects in the 12-minute sessions studied at the University of Massachusetts, both groups lost bodyfat. So for best results interval training sessions of 30 minutes or longer are recommended.

More Fun

"Another plus," says the *Wellness Letter,* "is that interval training is less monotonous than steady-pace exercise." I've found that this is true. As an example, five minutes on the Air-Dyne passes faster if I ride one minute at a load level of 6, one minute at 4, and three minutes at 5, as opposed to simply holding the resistance steady at 5. The average load, of course, is the same, but it seems easier, and it's more enjoyable when I vary the pace. Try this yourself; you'll see what I mean.

Finally, it's easy to set up a full interval training session. You can use almost any aerobic exercise, including the machines you mentioned. Thirty minutes (plus warm-up and cool-down) is a good workout length. Repetitions and recovery intervals can be of many different times, but in general it's best to alternate 15 seconds to three minutes of high-intensity work with low-intensity intervals of about the same length. Obviously, short intervals can be more intense than long ones. You'll also find that long repetition intervals require proportionately shorter recovery intervals. This is because it doesn't take as long, relatively speaking, to recover from longer, but less intense, work periods. The repetitions should get your heart rate up to 85-90% of maximum, and you shouldn't let your heart rate drop below 60% of maximum during "rest" intervals.

SWIM, WALK OR JOG FAT OFF?

Q: *After reading* Ripped 2, *I changed my diet and added aerobics to speed up my fat loss. I swim three times a week and jog twice a week. I also walk regularly. I've already lost 10 pounds and taken 2 inches off my waist. Although I'm pleased with my results, I have one concern.*

Covert Bailey's book Fit or Fat? *states that swimming causes your body to conserve fat. I like to swim, but I'd hate to think that swimming was slowing down my fat loss. What about this?*

A: After receiving your letter, I pulled out my dogeared copy of *Fit or Fat?* (Houghton Mifflin, 1977). (As you probably know, this wonderful little book — it's still a best seller — convinced me that I should increase my aerobic activity. *Fit or Fat?* is a must read for anyone interested in fat loss.) Bailey says that swimming is a great aerobic exercise, but he doesn't recommend it if you're overweight. "The swimmer's body," he explains, "tends to conserve its fat in order to provide warmth and buoyancy during the exercise." He states that swimming doesn't reduce bodyfat. Actually, there's recent evidence that swimming may encourage the addition of bodyfat.

Swimmers Gained!

Tufts University Diet & Nutrition Letter (April 1989) tells about recent research performed at the University of California, Irvine Medical Center. In a six-month exercise program three groups of overweight women either walked, cycled or swam. The walkers lost an average of 17 pounds, the cyclists 19 pounds, but the swimmers *gained* an average of 5 pounds each. How come?

Grant Gwinup, MD, the researcher who monitored the women, speculates that swimmers compensate for the calories they burn by eating more. *Diet & Nutrition Letter* summed up the doctor's reasoning this way: "Water draws much more heat away from the body than air, and swimmers' bodies sense that extra heat loss." This stimulates the swimmers' appetites so they'll eat more and hold on to the layers of fat that serve as heat-preserving insulation.

Bolstering this theory, the *Tufts Letter* points out that Polynesians, who are in the water a lot, are fatter on the whole than many other ethnic groups. Japanese women pearl divers, who spend hours on end in the sea, have also been found to be physically fit but fat. Bailey adds that sea mammals such as whales, seals and otters have large amounts of fat insulating their very well-trained muscles.

Walking For Weight Control

You are making good progress — lost inches on the waistline are solid evidence of fat loss — but if your progress slows, you might want

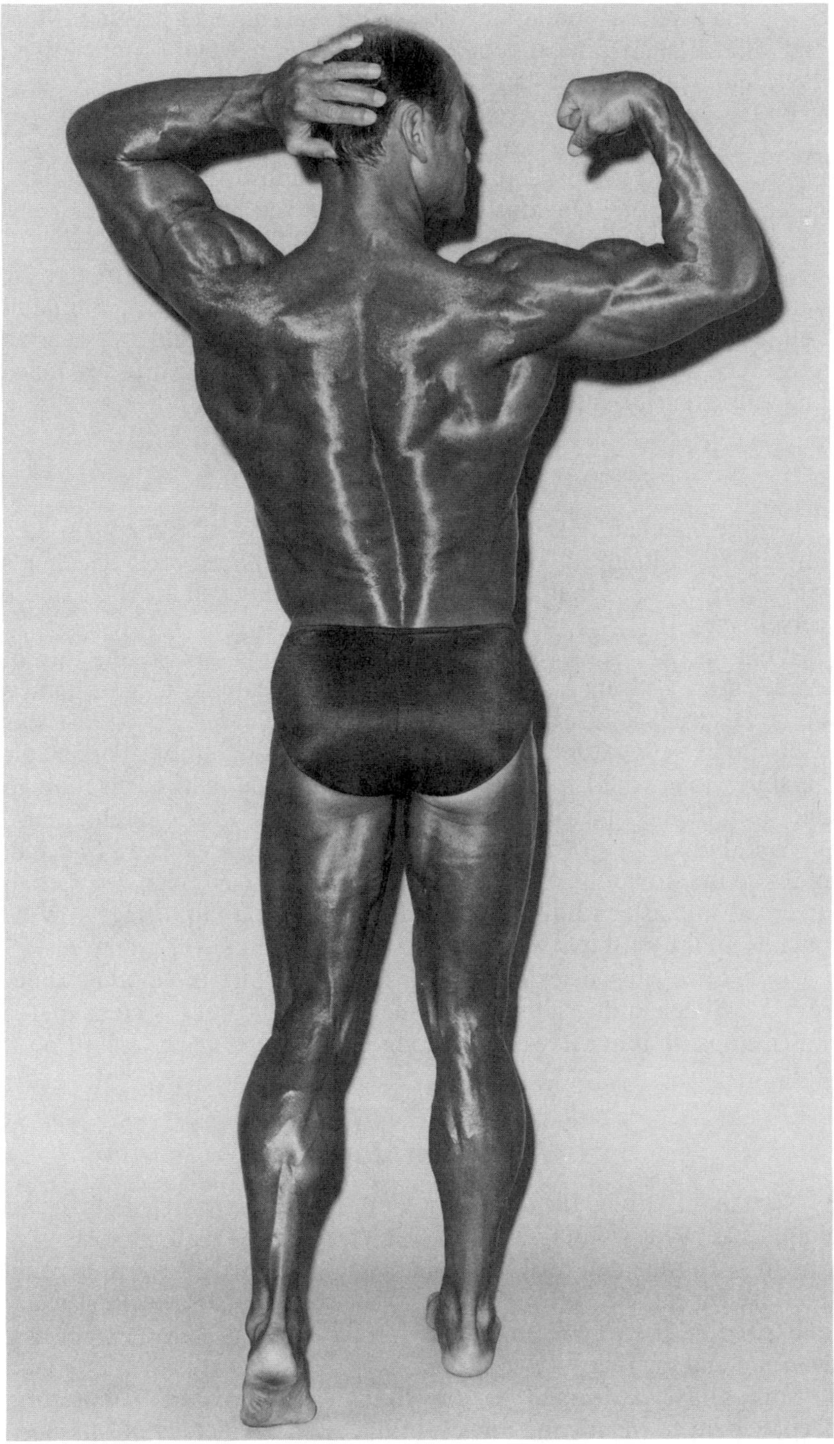

Photo by Dave Sauer.

to cut back on swimming and add more walking and jogging. More and more fitness-minded people are walking for weight control these days, and with good reason.

Bailey says if he were grossly fat, he'd walk three or four hours per day. This makes sense, because only a low-intensity exercise like walking will allow you to keep going long enough to burn a substantial number of calories. Obviously, you can walk further than you can run. "That's the crux of the matter," says the *Tufts University Diet & Nutrition Letter*, "because the greater the distance covered, the greater the number of calories used." For example, someone who walks a mile or two will burn far more calories overall than he would by wearing himself out running just a few blocks. For fat-burning purposes, duration, not intensity, is the key.

Poor Pultz

George Sheehan, MD, told a great story recently in "Running Wild," his regular column in *The Physician and Sportsmedicine*. Sheehan's tale of Pultz shows that simply walking every day can make an obese person lean.

What had first seemed an unfortunate and even devastating turn of events literally transformed his sister's letter carrier, a man named Pultz. His truck was taken away. In Sheehan's words, "Poor Pultz was overweight — his stomach hung over his belt, and buttons popped off his shirt. How would he ever negotiate the hills that marked his route to and from the post office? Everyone thought Pultz was through."

Well, I'm sure you've already guessed the happy outcome. Sheehan picks up the story four years later: "Pultz is now fit and lean. He used to arrive at my sister's house at 4:00 P.M. huffing and puffing; now he pounds up the path two hours early — an athlete delivering the mail."

Now, Sheehan's sister has a new concern: Pultz is thinking about retiring! Sheehan doesn't say how the story ends, but it's clear that if Pultz stops walking it won't be long before he is once again "poor Pultz."

Walking vs. Jogging

Now that I've beat the drums for walking, let me reverse course and emphasize what walking by itself won't do. While I walk almost every day to keep sane and lean, walking is not necessarily the best aerobic exercise for fat loss. Why is shown in the results of an excellent study published in *The Physician & Sportsmedicine* (May 1989) comparing walking and jogging.

This study, performed at the Human Performance Laboratory, Department of Health and Physical Education, University of Missouri, Columbia, compares the energy expended during prolonged walking and jogging. The unique feature is that the research is structured so that the exercise heart rate is the same for the walkers and the joggers. This is important because jogging usually produces a faster heart rate than walking. Plus, jogging a mile at a comfrotable pace requires more energy than walking the same distance; research sets the energy expenditure of jogging at least 20% higher. The reason is that joggers lift their feet higher into the air than walkers; they travel up and down as well as forward. This extra motion causes joggers to burn more calories. This particular study addressed the question of whether the energy expenditure difference would persist if the walkers and joggers maintained the same heart rate. Here's what happened.

With some difficulty, the researchers adjusted treadmill speed and angle so that nine young men walked and jogged at 65% of their maximum heart rate (about 125 beats per minute) for 60 minutes and 75% maximum heart rate (about 145 beats per minute) for 45 minutes. As you can well imagine, the men had to walk at a good clip, 4.7 mph for 65% heart rate maximum and 4.8 mph on a 3.6% incline for 75% heart rate maximum. Needless to say, the men found it more comfortable to achieve 65% and 75% maximum heart rate by jogging.

Even at the same heart rate, the joggers still burned substantially more calories: 4.7% and 7.5% more at 65% and 75% heart rate maximums, respectively. Significantly, the joggers also burned more fat calories.

At 65% heart rate maximum, the amount of fat used was 11.4% more during jogging than walking; at 75% heart rate maximum, the fat used was 21.2% more during jogging.

This is quite surprising because, as I implied earlier, fat use has been shown to be inversely related to exercise intensity. The University of Missouri researchers had a logical explanation. They said that previous work in their laboratory indicated that the degree of fat metabolism depends on the amount of muscle mass involved in the exercise. "The greater amount of muscle mass used during jogging vs. walking may produce a lower relative intensity of exercise per gram of muscle used." In other words, jogging spreads the stress over more of the body; individual muscle cells are actually under less stress.

Whole-Body Aerobics

I'll buy that. That's the reason I recommend whole-body aerobic exercise. Stationary bicycles with push-pull arm action, rowing machines that work the legs, cross country ski-machines and the HeavyHands system work both the upper and lower body; they allow you to burn more calories and more fat with less perceived effort.

What I've told you really boils down to a few simple points. Swimming is a great aerobic exercise. It'll make you fit, but it should not be the cornerstone of your program if you're overweight. Walking is a pleasant and comfortable way to burn a few extra calories every day. Over the weeks and months it really adds up. It's estimated that a 150-pound person who walks briskly for 45 minutes four times a week will burn enough calories to lose 18 pounds over the course of a year. Nevertheless, if you're fit enough you can burn substantially more calories and more fat by jogging. Even better, however, are aerobic exercises that use your torso, your arms and your legs. Whole-body aerobic exercise burns maximum fat in minimum time.

I wish you continued success. Whatever you do, enjoy it.

CROSS-TRAINING

Make every muscle a better fat burner

Q: *I'm a competitive triathlete with a keen interest in bodybuilding. What do you think about cross-training (combining several different aerobic activities) for bodybuilders?*

A: Whether cross-training improves performance in a specific sport is still an open question. The great debate continues whether biking, swimming or other aerobic alternatives will make you a better runner. No matter how this comes down, in my view, cross-training is ideal for bodybuilders. In terms of overall fitness, top-class triathletes are some of the best-conditioned athletes in the world. And as we've all observed from watching them on television, triathletes are also among the leanest of athletes. All bodybuilders want to be leaner and fitter, but without it interfering with their weight training. Cross-training fills the bill in both regards.

Two Systems

The first thing to keep in mind is that aerobic exercise produces a training effect in two different systems: the central and the peripheral. The central system is the heart and lungs. The peripheral system is the specific muscles being used.

All aerobic exercise stresses the central system. The heart and lungs can't tell what exercise is being performed. How hard the central system works is determined by the intensity of the exercise and the amount of muscle mass used to perform the activity.

Peripheral training effect is the adaptation that takes place in the actual muscles being used. A specific aerobic mechanism exists within each individual muscle. Aerobic exercise makes each muscle cell involved a more efficient oxygen-processing, glycogen-storing and *fat-burning* unit.

Working Muscles Benefit

The crucial point is that this training effect takes place only in the muscle fibers being used. For example, running and biking, according to biomechanist Peter Cavanagh, Ph.D., of Pennsylvania State University, "are radically different types of activities." Running makes the hamstrings and calves stronger, more durable and more efficient, while biking primarily affects the quadriceps. Both activities leave the muscles of the upper body relatively unaffected. By contrast, cross-country skiing, with its poling action, produces a training effect in both the upper and lower body. That's why cross-country skiers are generally considered to be the most aerobically fit of all athletes; they have total-body fitness.

Bodybuilders use aerobic exercise to reduce their bodyfat level. The energy for aerobic exercise comes mainly from fat. Aerobic exercise stimulates the production of enzymes that convert fat to energy. Those fat-burning enzymes are developed in the specific muscles being exercised.

It stands to reason, therefore, that a bodybuilder will benefit from conditioning all of his or her muscles aerobically. What better way to do that than through a combination of aerobic activities that, taken together, stimulate all or most of the muscles of the body? Maybe runners should run, run, run; cyclists should bike, bike, bike; and swimmers should swim, swim, swim; but bodybuilders, like triathletes, can clearly benefit from doing it all. With cross-training every muscle will burn fat most efficiently.

Total Body Conditioning

And there's more. Runner-writer-cardiologist George Sheehan reported recently in *Runner's World* that a study from Pennsylvania State University suggests that combination training does in fact improve performance in each individual activity. In this study, runners who added aerobic arm training to their program showed a delay in the onset of blood lactate accumulation. They also had lower peak lactate levels and a 35% quicker return to normal values during active recovery. Explained Sheehan, "Apparently these trained arm muscles had an increased ability to lower blood lactate."

Upper body training makes it possible for them to run at a faster pace without developing an oxygen debt, which precipitates a buildup of lactic acid. To use Sheehan's phrase, it gave them a higher "maximum cruising speed." This would be a plus for bodybuilders as well. It would allow them to train aerobically at a higher intensity level. Total body conditioning would allow them to burn more calories and more fat in a shorter period of time. In other words, with the higher cruising speed or anaerobic threshold developed through cross-training, you can devote less time to aerobics, leaving more time for the weights.

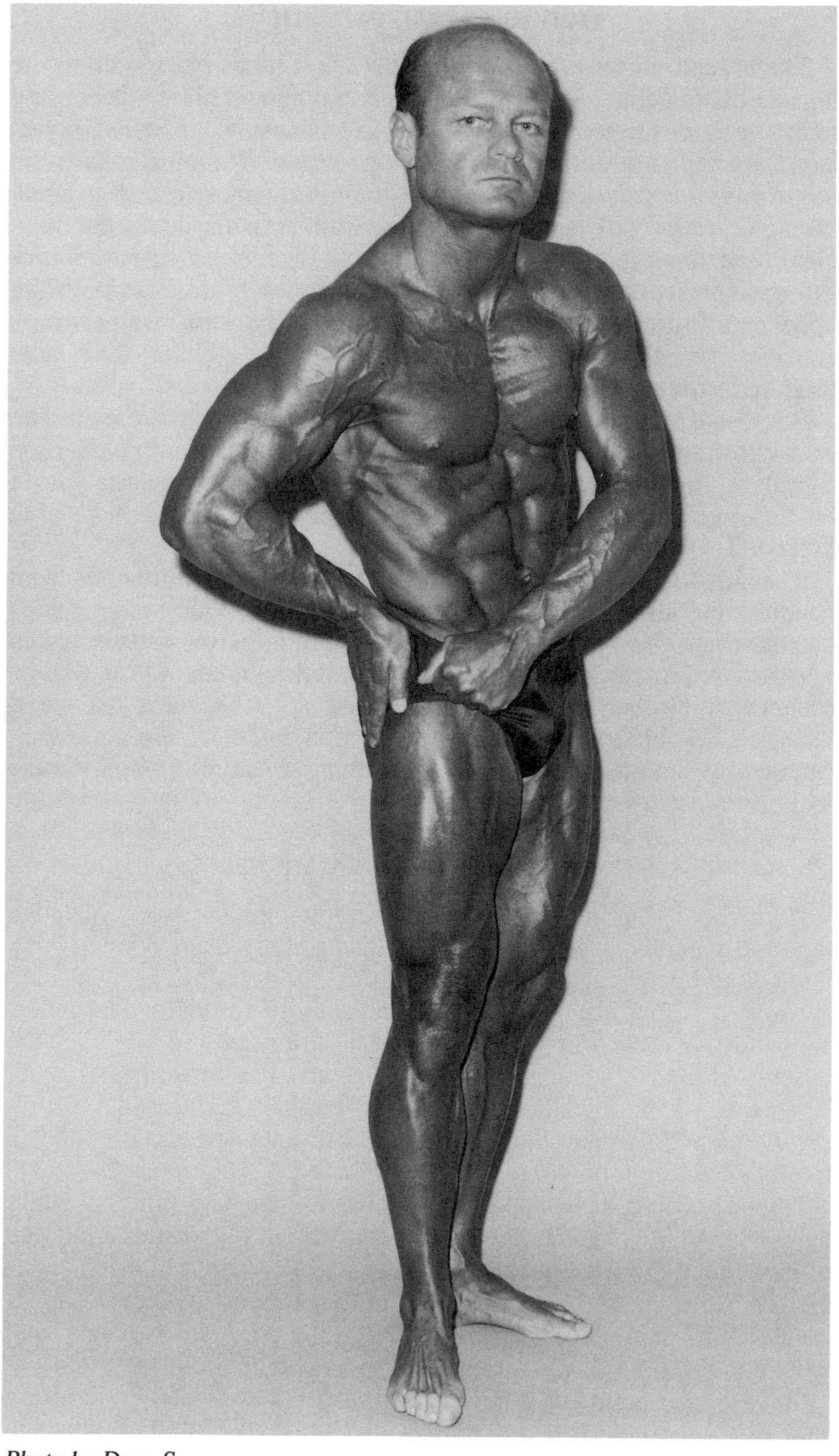

Photo by Dave Sauer.

Avoid Over-Training

This of course goes hand in hand with another benefit of cross-training on which everybody agrees. By combining several different activities, you can exercise more and harder without breaking down. The *University of California, Berkeley Wellness Letter* put it this way: "Over-training on one sport or activity continually stresses the same muscles and joints, thus increasing the risk of injury. If instead of running every day, you alternated it with swimming every other day, you'll give your leg muscles and joints a needed rest between runs." That's another advantage of combining several different types of exercise. Simply put, by varying your aerobic activities you can tolerate more volume and burn more fat. And moving the stress of aerobic exercise to different parts of the body leaves all the bodyparts fresher for weight sessions.

You're a competitive triathlete and a bodybuilder, so I assume you've already figured out how to fit these multiple activities into your schedule. To other bodybuilders, however, it may appear to be a mighty tight squeeze. Actually, as I've already indicated, cross-training makes it easier for a bodybuilder to include aerobic exercise in his or her program. To illustrate, I'll tell you how I used cross-training to prepare to return to the Cooper Clinic for retesting this past year. Combining cross-training with my regular bodybuilding program was easy. And it worked like a charm.

My main objective was to improve my time on the treadmill. As you may know, the angle of the treadmill increases 1% each minute to 25%, then the speed goes up 0.2 mph until exhaustion. Obviously, I had to get my climbing muscles in shape. Still, I didn't want to stress the same muscles and joints so much that it would interfere with weight training exercises like the squat. Cross-training did the job perfectly; it allowed me to do hard and frequent aerobic training without becoming overtrained.

Cross-Training Routine

In addition to my regular weight training program, I did aerobics three times a week. I didn't need more frequent sessions because alternating a climbing with a biking activity allowed me to train at high intensity every session. I should qualify that by explaining that I varied the intensity in coordination with my periodized weight training program. I increased the intensity in phases. I started each phase easy and built to a peak in the fourth or fifth week. Then I started the process over again. I tried to build to a higher peak at the end of each phase. (See my book *Ripped 3* for a complete explanation of periodization for bodybuilders.)

I used two climbing activities — the treadmill and climbing the mountain trail near my home — and two biking activities — my regular bicycle outdoors, and indoors the Schwinn Air-Dyne stationary bicycle with a push-pull arm action. I scheduled my hardest aerobic workouts on Sunday, climbing and biking in alternation. On the other two aerobic sessions each week I also alternated climbing and biking. My weekday sessions were easier, but still relatively intense. In addition, I burned a few more calories and speeded my recovery by walking at least 30 minutes almost every day.

A typical two-week schedule went something like this:

Sunday — Climb mountain
Tuesday — Air-Dyne
Thursday — Treadmill
Sunday — Outdoor bike
Tuesday — Treadmill
Thursday — Air-Dyne
Sunday — Climb mountain

My Sunday workouts took about an hour including warm-up and cool-down, and the weekday sessions were about 45 minutes.

You'll note that even though better treadmill performance was my main training objective, I still trained on the treadmill only once a week. As the actual test approached, I did schedule the treadmill on Sundays occasionally. Even then, however, I avoided doing the treadmill hard more than once a week.

I'm convinced that this worked better than training on the treadmill all the time. I know it was more fun. Training on the treadmill alone would have been boring. I would have grown to hate the treadmill. This combination of activities kept both my mind and body fresh. The results show it also prepared me well for my rematch with the Cooper Clinic treadmill.

Fitness Payoff

I lasted 29 minutes, beating my previous time by a full minute! This placed me 2½ minutes above the 99th percentile for the 50-59 age group. It also put me well into the superior category, the top group, for men under 30. And I'm in my early 50s!

I think I proved that cross-training is a good way to prepare for a treadmill test. My guess is that cross-training will improve one's performance in any sport where fitness and leanness are important. That includes bodybuilding. So my advice is to keep doing what you're doing.

WALKING TO THE PEAK

Get camera-ready with walking

Strangers who see me out walking might well say: "Look at that old coot. He's too old, too lazy or too out-of-shape to do anything else." People tend to think of walking as a casual, beginning-level fitness activity. It is that, of course. I see walking in another light, however. It can play an important role in a carefully designed bodybuilding program. I'll use my own example to illustrate how walking can aid a bodybuilder.

Invitation From Weider

When *Muscle & Fitness* Executive Editor Mary Ann Mucica invited me to California recently for some photos, I made only two changes in my training program. I reduced my daily food intake by about 150 calories and I added about 30 minutes of daily walking to my exercise program. Let me explain why I was willing to rely on these seemingly minor alterations to get ready for something as important as a photo session for Joe Weider.

I already had a good exercise program in place, weights and aerobics. My diet was well under control; I was taking in about 2,600 calories a day. The Futrex-5000 Body Fat Computer said my bodyfat was 5%, and the mirror confirmed that I was already relatively lean. A few simple calculations showed that shedding about 3 pounds of fat would get me down to 3% bodyfat, where I look best.

The easiest and most comfortable way to accomplish that reduction, I knew from past experience, would be walking. Why not simply cut calories more than 150 per day? I decided not to do that for two reasons. First, if I ate less I'd make myself hungry and uncomfortable. Psychologically, that's a mistake. As I've said before, you almost always compensate by bingeing. In the long run, you end up fatter than ever.

Secondly, severe calorie restriction is also a mistake from the physiological standpoint. As Covert Bailey said in his fat-loss classic *Fit or Fat?* (Houghton Mifflin, 1977), severe calorie restriction encourages your body to become fatter. Research has proven, he explained, that severe diets cause the body to produce more of the enzymes responsible for the depositing of fat. These fat-depositing enzymes create what Bailey called "a fat person's chemistry." They create a tendency to get fat.

Learning From Experience

I can tell you from personal experience that Bailey is correct. In the

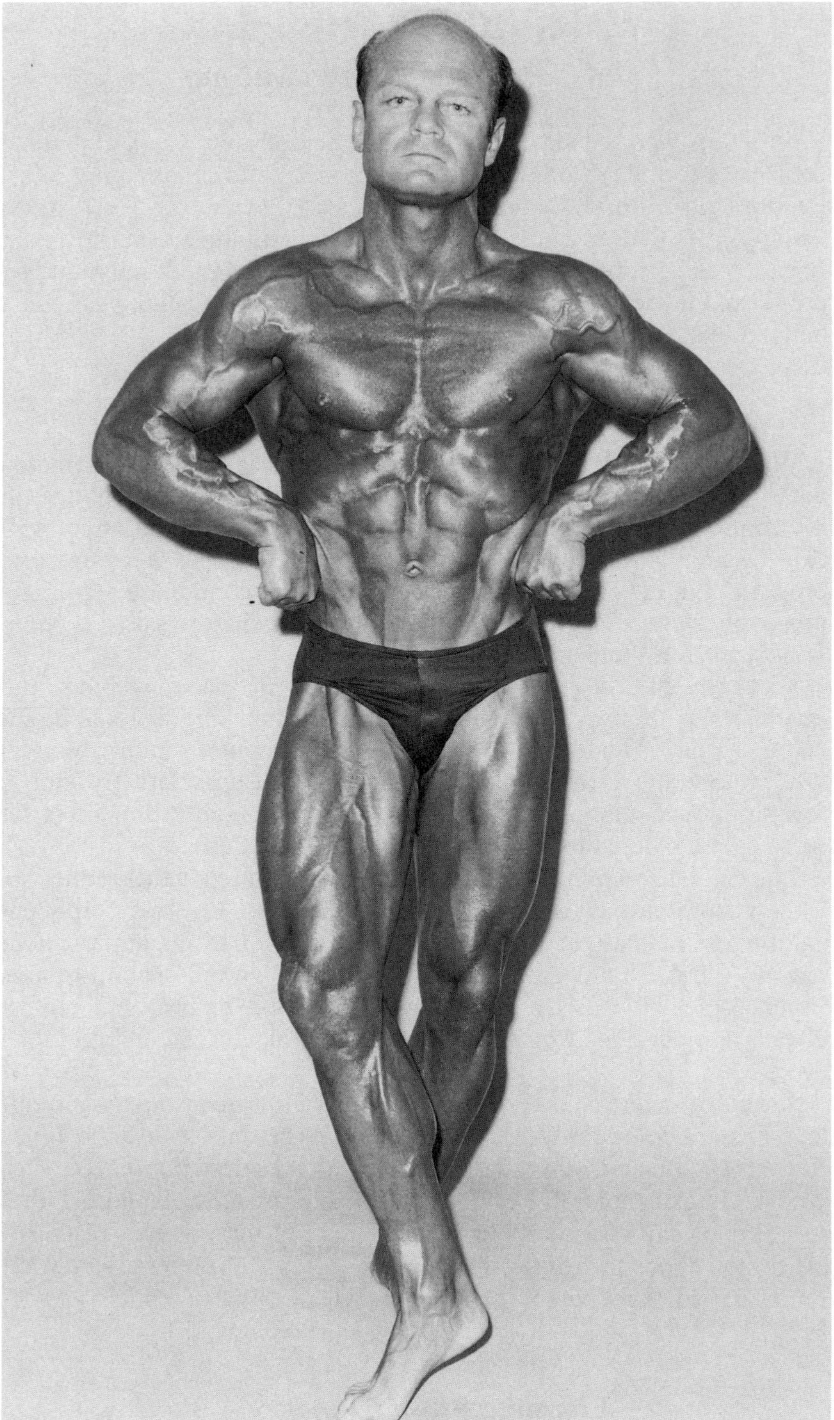

Photo by Dave Sauer.

past, I've cut back too much on calories only to find myself getting fatter. I lost weight all right, but I *gained* fat. How about doing more sets and reps with the weights to burn more calories and shed the excess fat? That would be a mistake as well. Weight training is anaerobic (without oxygen) exercise. It requires short bursts of high-intensity effort. The energy for this type of stop-and-go exercise comes from glycogen, a carbohydrate, stored in the muscles. Weight training burns almost no fat, because fat can't be converted to energy fast enough. Longer term, weight training is important, because it builds and maintains calorie-burning muscle tissue.

That brings us to aerobic (with oxygen) exercise which, by definition, is low-intensity effort that can be continued for a long period of time. The energy for aerobic exercise comes mainly from fat. That's what I needed. Still, as noted, aerobic exercise was already a part of my program.

Why Walking?

It wouldn't do to add more rowing, biking, running or similar activities. These are all relatively intense forms of aerobic exercise; I don't like to do them more often than every two or three days. That's because, in addition to burning fat, they deplete the glycogen stored in your muscles. As Lawrence E. Lamb, MD, said in *The Weighting Game* (Lyle Stuart, 1988), if your glycogen stores are depleted, you will not have the energy to work your muscles. It may take two or three days to replenish a muscle with glycogen, Lamb explained. Doing more of this type of aerobic exercise would keep my muscles in a state of fatigue. I wouldn't be able to do justice to my weight-training program. (Again, longer term, intense forms of aerobic exercise are important, because they train the muscles to burn fat more readily.) That, of course, leaves walking.

Exercise below 80% of your maximum heart rate is generally considered to be aerobic. As I've already said, the energy for aerobic exercise comes mainly from fat. Nevertheless, some glycogen is burned even during aerobic exercise. In general, the milder the exercise, the greater the proportion of fat burned. Walking is extremely aerobic, because it keeps your heart rate well under 80% of maximum. It comes about as close as anything can to being a pure fat-burning activity.

Emphasizing this in *Fit or Fat?*, Covert Bailey wrote: "If I were grossly fat, I would give up whatever is necessary — job, housework, whatever — and would walk three to four hours per day."

That's a bit extreme, but it illustrates why I chose walking to help me prepare for the photo session with Joe Weider. Walking a little extra each day will burn off the few pounds of fat I need to lose. The average-sized person burns about 150 calories walking 30 minutes; combined with a 150-calorie dietary reduction, that works out to about two-thirds of a pound of fat each week. And it will do it without making me miserable or interfering with my regular weight and aerobic exercise program.

What's more, the gentle stimulation of walking will help my muscles unload waste products faster; that will speed my recovery from intense exercise sessions. In short, for a bodybuilder, walking is a win-win activity.

So, the next time you need to lose a few pounds of fat to hit your peak, try walking it off.

GAUGING FAT-BURNING PACE

Debunking the fat-burn zone

Many bodybuilders worry too much about heart rate when they do aerobic exercise. This came to my attention when I visited an old training partner during my recent trip to California. We lifted together about 25 years ago when he was in the Air Force stationed in Albuquerque.

Still in good shape — he had just entered an over-50 physique contest — he rides the Lifecycle as part of his regular workouts. As most of you know, the Lifecycle is a computerized exercise bike with different levels of intensity; Level 1 is the easiest and 12 the hardest. My old friend rides at Level 5 or 6, which is easy enough to allow him to read throughout the 24-minute Hill Program. I asked why he didn't push himself more. His answer: "I want to be sure my heart rate stays in the fat-burning range."

This subject came up again the next day, when Chris Lund photographed me at the extremely well-equipped Marina Athletic Club in Marina del Rey. One large room was given almost entirely to aerobic exercise equipment. The walls were lined with machines — you name it, they have it — practically all of which were in use. But what really caught my eye was this: About half of the people, like my old friend, were doing aerobic exercise... and reading!

Apparently people are confused about the pace that burns fat best. If you push too hard, it's true, you burn carbohydrate and not fat. Still, that doesn't mean you have to loaf along at a reading pace. It's only common sense that the faster you go, the more calories you burn. The problem is that if you push too hard, you can't continue long enough to burn very many calories. You get out of breath. The lactic acid builds up in your muscles and you simply can't continue.

Physiologically, your body can't process oxygen fast enough. That's what aerobic exercise is, exercise with oxygen. The body requires oxygen to burn fat. If you get ahead of your fat-burning capacity, the energy must come from glycogen, a carbohydrate stored in the muscles. Exercise at that level is called anaerobic, which means without oxygen.

Some experts, I know, recommend monitoring heart rate to stay at the aerobic level. But, in my view, that's more trouble than it's worth, and it's really not necessary. The fat-burn problem basically takes care of itself. Let me explain.

Maximum Heart Rate

As a rule of thumb, exercise below 80-85% of your maximum heart rate is aerobic and exercise above that is anaerobic. As a practical matter, however, this guideline doesn't work very well.

First, it's hard to determine your maximum heart rate unless you have a stress test done on a treadmill. You can, of course, use the standard formula that says your maximum heart rate is your age subtracted from 220. The problem is that this formula doesn't apply to everyone.

I'm one for whom the formula doesn't work. At age 53, my maximum heart rate should be 167 (220 minus 53 equals 167). It's not, however. Stress tests over the past 15 years have shown my maximum heart rate to be over 180. On the other hand, some people have a naturally slow heart rate. They can't get their heart rate up to the maximum called for by the formula. That's neither good nor bad; it's just the way it is.

Another problem, of course, is that it's difficult to take your exercising pulse accurately. In my experience, most pulse meters don't function well, and it's tricky trying to count your heart rate in the middle of an exercise session.

Another thing that confounds the formula is that aerobic exercise pace changes with fitness level. For example, a 5-minute-per-mile pace may be aerobic for a well-conditioned marathon runner. On the other hand, an out-of-shape individual may be unable to run a mile at any speed. For that person, anything faster than walking may be anaerobic. After a period of training, however, that same person may be able to run continuously at an 8-minute-per-mile pace, burning fat all the way. In other words, an individual's aerobic pace is a moving target.

Simple Guideline

What guideline can a bodybuilder use to ensure maximum fat-burning benefit from aerobic exercise? It's simple, really. William D. McArdle, Frank I. Katch and Victor L. Katch in their textbook *Exercise Physiology* (Lea & Febiger, 1986) state that anything beyond a one-half mile run is predominantly aerobic. Listen to what they say: "Prolonged exercise progresses on a 'pay-as-you-go' basis with more

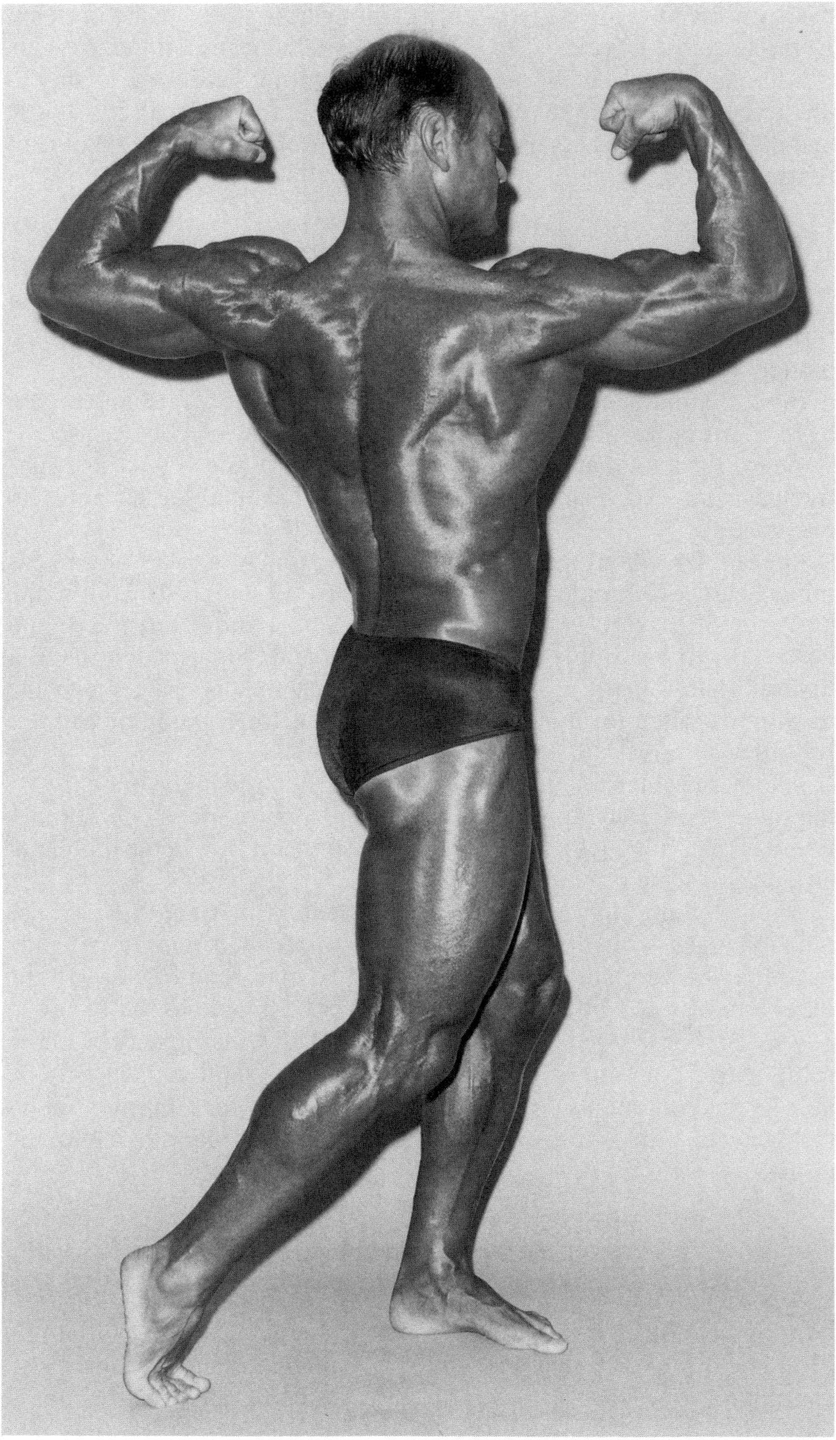

Photo by Dave Sauer.

than 99% of the energy requirement being generated by aerobic reactions." In short, any pace you can maintain for more than a few minutes burns mainly fat. So if your aerobic sessions last 20-30 minutes, you're safely in the fat-burn zone.

Covert Bailey and Lee Bishop give basically the same advice in their excellent book, *The Fit Or Fat Woman* (Houghton Miffln, 1989). Your degree of breathlessness while exercising for a sustained 15-20 minutes, they say, is a better indicator of aerobic pace than pulse. Then, using an imaginary conversation, they paint a word picture of correct pace.

While you're exercising, someone might ask, "Where are you from?" If all you can do is gasp, "Ohio," you're going too fast. On the other hand, if you rattle off, "I'm from Canton, Ohio. I live on West 63rd in a split-level, four-bedroom, 2,000-square-foot home with my husband, three kids, dog and a parakeet," you're not going fast enough. If you're right on aerobic pace, however, Bailey and Bishop say you'd answer like this: "I'm from Ohio — (pant, pant) — near the outskirts of Toledo — (pant, pant) — in a little farming community."

Aerobic Overload Training

Note that the Bailey and Bishop illustration includes a pace that's too slow. That's why I questioned my old training partner's riding/reading pace. If you can read, you're not getting optimum benefit from your aerobic sessions.

Just about every bodybuilder has heard of the Overload Principle, which says you have to make your muscles work harder than normal or they won't grow. Well, the same principle also applies to aerobic exercise. If you want the maximum fat-burning benefit from your aerobic sessions, then you must, at least occasionally, push harder than normal.

With aerobic overload training, explain McArdle and the Katches, "There is an increase in the trained muscle's capacity to mobilize and oxidize fat." That's important, because it means that with training you'll develop the capacity to burn more fat than an untrained person. In short, you'll get more fat-burning benefit if you put more effort into your aerobic exercise sessions.

So you see, there's no free lunch. Effective aerobics and reading really don't mix. Put on the headphones or turn up the TV, but save the newspaper for later. You can also skip the pulse meter.

A little experience is all that's required. Just set a pace that makes you work, but that can be maintained for 20 minutes or more. Exercise physiologists call this "perceived rate of exertion." Combined with common sense, it's all a bodybuilder needs to achieve maximum fat-burning benefit from aerobic exercise.

STAIR CLIMBING MACHINES

Is there magic in these popular devices?

Q: *What do you think about the stair climbers that are so popular these days? Are they good for burning calories and keeping lean and fit?*

A: I know the machines are in constant demand in health clubs. When I was photographed late last year at the well-equipped Marina Athletic Club in Marina del Rey, California, we had to wait until the second day of shooting to find a free stair climber. I've also tried a relative's home model stepper. The motion is great. I liked it so much that I'm thinking about getting a good quality climber for our home gym. With this in mind, I've done some research and thinking about stair machines. I'll tell you my conclusions.

Main Appeal

Besides the fact that they are relatively new on the scene, the main appeal of stair climbers is that they provide a lot of exercise in a short period of time. That's because they use the large muscles in the lower back, hips and legs. Because so much muscle mass is involved all at one time, more calories and fat are burned than with, for example, a stationary bike, which focuses the effort primarily on the quads.

Like any other exercise, however, you have to do it properly and work hard to get maximum benefit. For example, leaning on the armrests and taking short, choppy steps, like many people do, cuts down on the effectiveness of the exercise. For best results, keep the weight on your feet and take full-sized steps.

On the other hand, you also lessen the benefit by trying to get too much done too quickly. Don't make your stepper workout so intense that you can't keep going very long. It's like a 100-yard dash compared to running — or even walking — a mile. The dash may seem like more effort, but the mile walk or run actually burns more calories. So don't make your stairclimb workouts too intense. Remember also that short, maximum efforts are more apt to cause injury.

Easy On The Knees?

Some say that stair machines are easy on the knees, but that's not necessarily so. Dr. James M. Fox, a member of the Southern California Orthopedic Institute in Van Nuys and author of *Save Your Knees,* says that climbing stairs adds 4-6 times the weight of the body on the kneecap area and that may cause knee problems. Lawrence E. Lamb, MD, writing in *The Health Letter,* advises that individuals with bad knees would do better on a stationary bicycle.

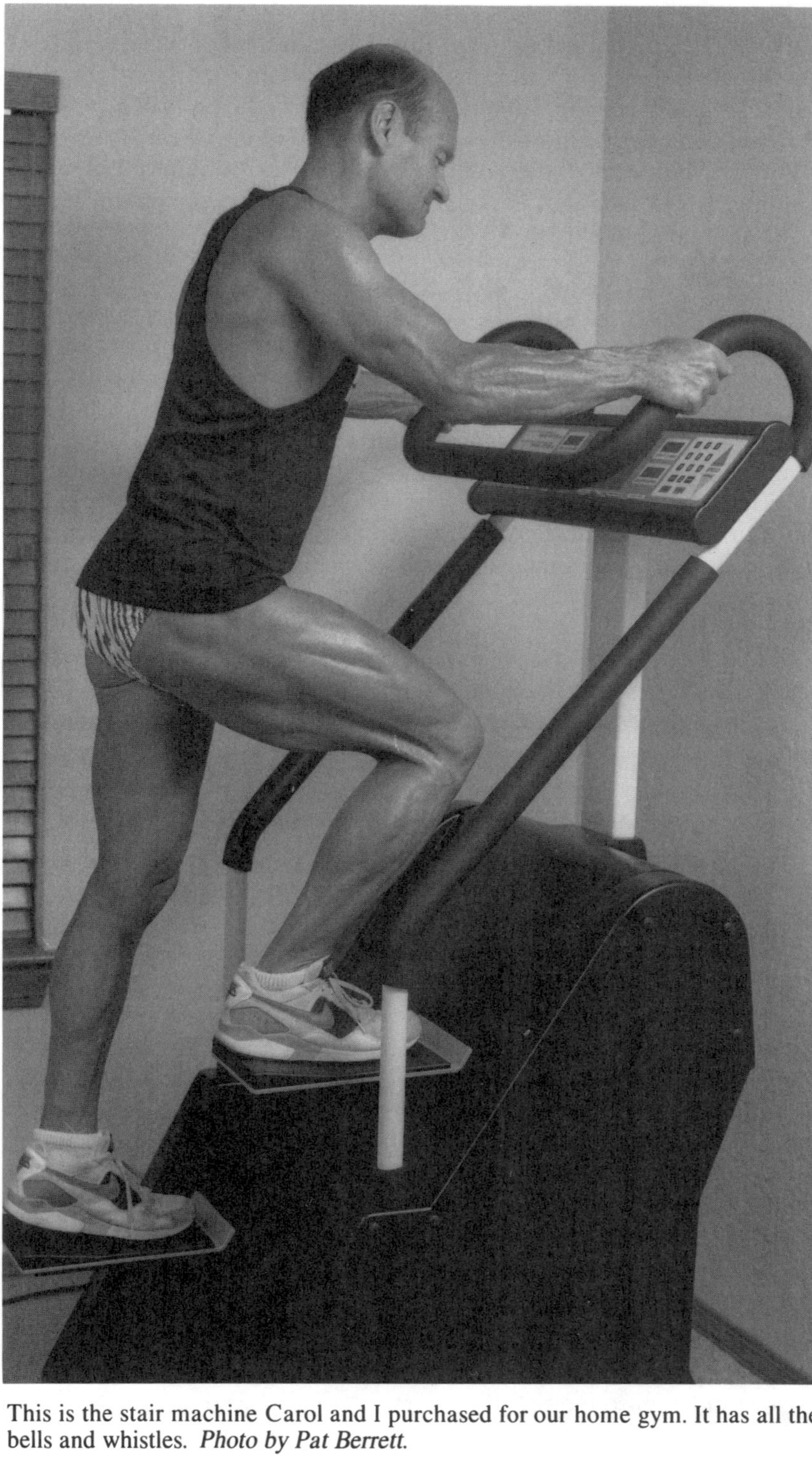

This is the stair machine Carol and I purchased for our home gym. It has all the bells and whistles. *Photo by Pat Berrett.*

My experience is that aches and pains crop up when you overdo any exercise. Even if your knees are fine, I recommend a wide variety of aerobic exercises. For example, it's better to alternate stair climbing and biking. This changes the points of stress on the body. The result is that you can tolerate more activity without breaking down. That's why Olympic Marathon gold medalist Frank Shorter combines biking and running. He's found that the combination makes it possible for him to exercise more and harder.

In The Muscles Themselves

Remember, too, that more than 50% of the benefit from aerobic exercise takes place within the muscles themselves. Aerobic exercise makes your muscle cells more efficient oxygen-processing and fat-burning units. It's only the involved muscles that benefit, however. So in addition to the stair climber, it's a good idea to do some aerobic exercise for the upper body as well. Take advantage of machines that work the muscles above your belt. The Versa Climber uses the arms as well as the legs, and some exercise bikes include a push-pull action for the arms. Rowing machines, of course, involve the pulling muscles of the upper body.

Some stair steppers have dual-action handlebars for upper body work. I haven't tried these, but the ones I've seen in sporting goods stores look promising. You get the idea. Spread the stress as widely as you can.

Computer Monitors Important

The flashy computer screens on many models of stair machines, showing information ranging from stairs climbed per minute to calories burned, also add to the appeal. People like the high-tech wizardry. I do too. The feedback offered by performance monitors is critical for motivation. If I buy a stepper, it will have the best computer monitor I can afford. That's because I know from experience that the added interest generated is worth the money.

That's not to say, of course, that the computer monitors are entirely accurate. Says James M. Rippe, MD, director of the Exercise Physiology and Nutrition Laboratory and associate professor of medicine at the University of Massachusetts Medical School in Worcester, "I have serious reservations as to whether those numbers have meaning." Rippe questions the computer-generated information on stair machines because it's based on what is known about the energy required to climb actual stairs. The biomechanics of the two activities may be different. Your bodyweight and composition and how closely you follow the computer program also affect accuracy. Nevertheless, the monitors are important because they allow you to compare workouts and measure progress.

The bottom line is that there's nothing magical about stair machines. I can get the same effect by climbing the mountain behind my house. Still, like most people, I enjoy new equipment. It adds spice to exercise, and that's important.

I recommend stair machines. Just be sure you also take advantage of the other equipment in the gym where you train. That includes, of course, the weights. No fitness program is complete without weight training.

If, like me, you're equipping a home gym, I suggest you purchase the best stepper your pocketbook permits.

MONITOR TO MOTIVATE

A change of heart on heart monitors

Q: *In response to your column "Gauging Fat-Burning Pace" in May, I wish to take issue with you regarding the effectiveness of heart rate monitors (HRMs) as an exercise tool.*

A little more than a year ago I was grossly overweight at 275 pounds with a cholesterol level of above 250 and a VO_2 max measured on a treadmill at 19 ml/kg min. I went on a medically monitored diet and in about five months I was down to 188 pounds with a cholesterol level of 135. Further tests showed my bodyfat to be 18.2% and that my VO_2 max had improved to 68.3.

Exercise, of course, contributed greatly to the quality of my weight loss. It made the loss mostly fat and was the main factor in improving my aerobic fitness. That's where the HRM comes in.

I became intrigued when I observed a heart monitor in operation during my treadmill test. I investigated and eventually bought an HRM distributed by Polar USA, Inc.; it's the chest-strap type and beeps when you go above or below your individual aerobic training zone.

In your books and columns, you encourage people to set goals and constantly challenge themselves. My HRM helped me do that. It showed that I had to work harder as my condition improved; my heart rate gradually declined as I became more trained. So I had to go faster to achieve the target zone. The monitor registered my progress in black and white; it proved to me that my training was working. So, you see, the HRM can be a worthwhile training tool.

A: Congratulations on your remarkable improvement. Your weight/fat loss is outstanding. (I'm glad you had a doctor to supervise your diet, because you lost faster than I normally recommend.) Your change in blood cholesterol level is wonderful as well, but I'm most impressed by the improvement in your VO_2 max. As indicated by the hospital report you enclosed, your aerobic fitness is now in the 99th percentile.

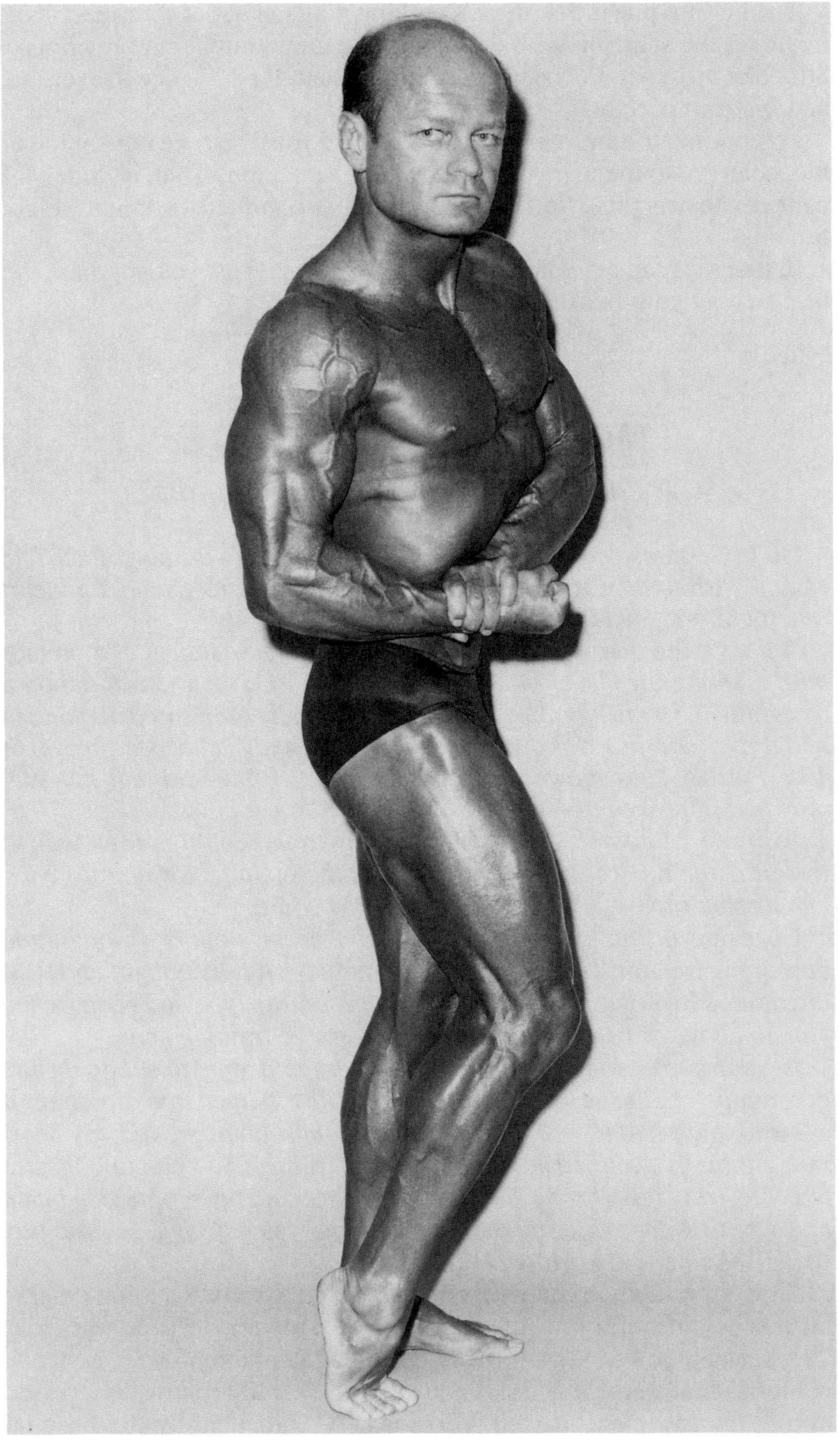

Photo by Dave Sauer.

You're right up there with world-class endurance athletes!

Past Experience

Your letter and some others I received prompted me to take another look at heart rate monitors. As explained in the earlier column, my experience has been that they don't work very well. I've owned a number of HRMs that clip to the ear lobe or the tip of the finger; I've also owned the baton type that you grasp with both hands. I stopped using them for the same reason I no longer rely on a training partner. It ruins the workout when your training partner doesn't show up; likewise, it's a downer when your HRM malfunctions in the middle of a training session.

With experience, I learned it was just as easy — and a lot more reliable — to use "perceived rate of exertion," or my own gut sense of how hard I'm working. As the American College of Sports Medicine says, as long as I exercise "somewhat hard" to "hard," I know I'll get significant aerobic benefit — and burn mainly fat as well.

New Research

Nevertheless, research after receiving your letter tells me that HRMs have improved. *U.S. News & World Report* magazine had Georgetown University test the current crop. In a 95-minute test, 16 monitors were simultaneously matched against an $18,000, 12-lead electrocardiogram (ECG). The new chest-strap monitors were found to be the most accurate. One, the $249 Polar Accurex, which I assume is the one you have, was "flawless." Its heart-rate readings coincided exactly with the ECG.

As you suggest, these new monitors let you punch in your own training zone, based on your individual heart rate maximum and fitness level. You can have your maximum heart rate measured on a treadmill, or you can estimate it using the standard formula: your age subtracted from 220.

According to the American College of Sports Medicine, the optimum training zone is 60-90% of your HR max. Below the minimum intensity level you're still burning fat, but you won't see much improvement in aerobic capacity. If you exceed the ceiling threshold, you'll develop an oxygen debt, lactic acid will build up and you'll soon be forced to stop or slow down. (Better-conditioned athletes may want to use a slightly tougher formula developed by the Cooper Clinic in Dallas: subtract half your age from 205 to find your theoretical maximum, and then multiple by .65 and .8.)

Valuable Feedback

In the previous column, I emphasized the need for aerobic overload. As you become fitter, you have to run, cycle, row or whatever harder to get your heart rate up to the training zone. People sometimes overlook this important point. In fact, they use the aerobic training zone concept as an excuse to slack off. Your example illustrates, however, that a reliable HRM actually helps you guard against this. It provides feedback that reminds you to continually up the ante, that is, if you want to keep improving.

In sum, you've convinced me that the new-and-improved heart rate monitors can be a valuable fitness tool. Success is what makes training enjoyable — it's also what keeps you motivated — and anything that documents success is worthwhile.

My order for a Polar Accurex is in the mail. Thanks for the tip.

PULSE MONITOR ONE YEAR LATER

Chest-strap devices deliver precision workout info

Q: *In the November 1991* M&F *(Monitor To Motivate) you wrote that recent research had persuaded you to take another look at heart-rate monitors (HRMs). You decided to order one of the new chest-strap monitors, a Polar Accurex. More than a year has passed. What has been your experience with it?*

A: As I stated in the earlier column, I've owned a number of the ear-, finger- and baton-type monitors and found that they had a maddening tendency to malfunction in the middle of a training session. I gave up on them some years back and came to rely on "perceived rate of exertion," or my own gut sense of how hard I'm working. I relented, however, after reading in *U.S. News & World Report* that Georgetown University had tested the current crop of HRMs and found the new chest-strap monitors to be more accurate than the older versions. In particular, the Polar Accurex, to which you refer, gave readings that coincided exactly with an $18,000 electrocardiogram (ECG).

That did it. I placed my order post-haste. And I'm glad I did. The only problem I've had is that electrical interference from my Lifecycle and stair machine causes the monitor to give off-the-wall readings. But for all other aerobic workouts, my Polar Accurex works just as the Georgetown researchers reported: flawlessly.

What's more, it turns out that my Polar unit is excellent for monitoring waking heart rate. Most doctors and exercise physiologists say the best time to check resting heart rate is when you wake up in the morning. At other times during the day, outside influences make it difficult to accurately gauge your heart rate at rest.

It's helpful to monitor your resting pulse, because it indicates whether or not you are recovering between workouts. Once you know your resting heart rate — well-trained athletes average about 50 beats per minute at rest, and sedentary individuals are usually about 20 beats higher — you can spot an elevated heart rate by checking yourself first thing in the morning. If your waking heart rate is five beats or more faster than normal, that usually means you have not recovered and should consider taking an easy workout that day — or simply rest.

Finally, An Accurate Reading

Like having a physiologist by your bed

I've never had much success taking my waking pulse manually on my wrist or neck. I seem to either fall asleep in the middle of the count or get so stirred up in the process that my heart speeds up before I can get an accurate reading. So I was delighted to find that the chest-strap monitor makes it easy. I go to the bathroom when I wake up and then put on the monitor before returning to bed. I lie down and relax for a few minutes, and when I open my eyes, it's right in front of me: my resting heart rate clearly displayed on the wrist receiver.

I never dreamed it could be so simple. It's almost like having an exercise physiologist by the bed to check my heart rate each morning. (The newly introduced Polar Favor HRM also works well for this purpose. It sells for $119 and turns on and off automatically, with no buttons to push when you're only half awake. The drawback to this model is that it has no memory function and cannot be programmed to record when you fall above or below your training zone.)

Changes in resting heart rate also reflect improved cardiovascular condition. As indicated above, training lowers resting heart rate. According to *Exercise Physiology* (Lea & Febiger, 1991), the excellent text by William D. McArdle, Frank I. Katch and Victor L. Katch, the heart muscle strengthened through training is capable of a more forceful stroke with each contraction. The result is that the heart does the same work while beating at a slower rate. Happily, most sedentary individuals experience a reduction in resting heart rate after only a few weeks of training. A good HRM shows the progress in black and white. Needless to say, that's very encouraging.

An HRM can also measure improvement from workout to workout. That's because your heart rate tells you how hard you're working, so it provides a convenient index to measure training improvement. For example, at the start of training your heart may beat 150 times per minute while you are running at a 10-minute-mile pace. After a period of conditioning, however, you'll probably be able to run at an eight-minute-mile pace with the same or slower heart rate. A heart-rate monitor registers your fitness advance and, again, that's very satisfying.

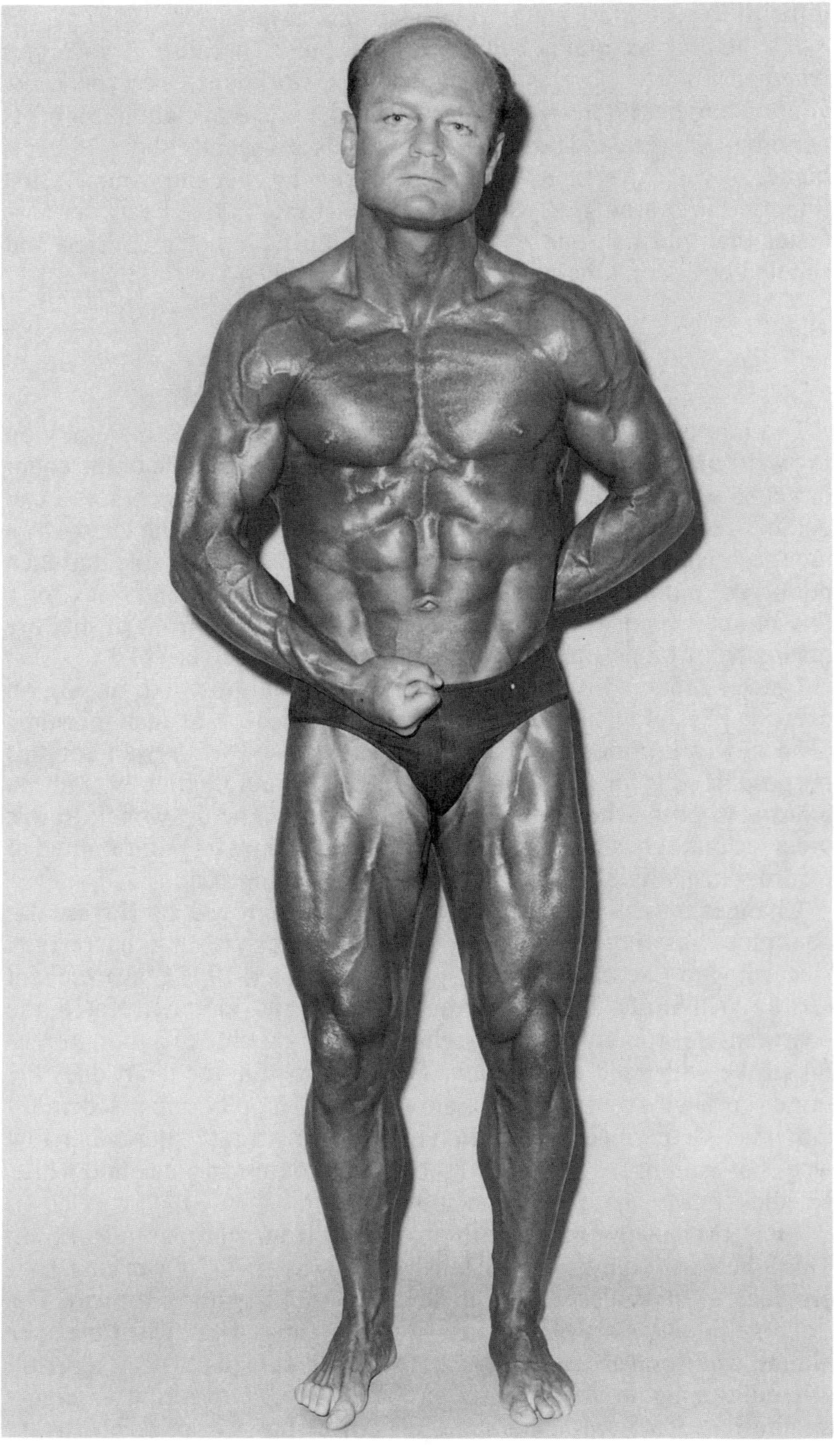

Photo by Dave Sauer.

Getting The Most From Your HRM

How to chart your improvement

It's important to realize, however, that heart rate varies with different forms of exercise. For example, McArdle and his colleagues point out that in both trained and untrained subjects the maximum heart rate while swimming and other forms of arm exercise averages about 10-13 beats per minute lower than the average heart rate while running. Body position, the muscle groups exercised, whether the exercise is continuous or stop-and-go and many other factors influence heart rate. This means one shouldn't try to compare the strenuousness of different activities — aerobic dance and circuit weight training, for example — on the basis of heart rate. In other words, be sure you are comparing apples and apples, not apples and oranges.

Some examples from my own training may help clarify this point. Most experts say aerobic capacity improves when you train between 60-90% of your maximum heart rate. In keeping with this rule of thumb, I've programmed my Accurex for a training zone from 110-165 beats per minute. It records my time above, below and within this heartbeat range. For example, in a recent treadmill workout the monitor showed that I spent eight minutes and 50 seconds above my target zone, 21 minutes and 30 seconds within the zone, and five minutes below. That was an improvement, because the last time I did the same treadmill workout, I spent nine minutes and 20 seconds above the target zone.

In short, the HRM says I did this workout with less effort than before; my heart didn't have to work as hard. (In case you're wondering, no definitive research exists that proves or disproves the value of training above 90% of heart-rate maximum. Generally, however, highly trained individuals need high intensity to make gains. According to my HRM, I spend some time above the usually recommended training zone in most aerobic workouts.)

Similarly, in a rowing workout of about the same duration, the monitor recorded that I spent five minutes at a heart rate above 165 beats per minute. A few weeks later I repeated the same workout, but this time with only three minutes and 10 seconds above my training zone. So once again, my condition improved. Note, however, that these readings do not provide a basis for comparing the relative intensity of my treadmill and rowing workouts. That would not be a valid comparison. My guess is that the maximum heart rate for rowing, like swimming, is lower than for treadmill training. Loose comparisons based on heart rate would probably underestimate the difficulty of rowing sessions.

In sum, I've found my new HRM to be a reliable training aid. Used properly — to compare apples and apples — it's a powerful motivator. Frankly, after a workout, I can hardly wait to check to see if I've improved. Yes, I love my chest-strap monitor.

CHAPTER SEVEN

PHYSIOLOGICAL FACTORS

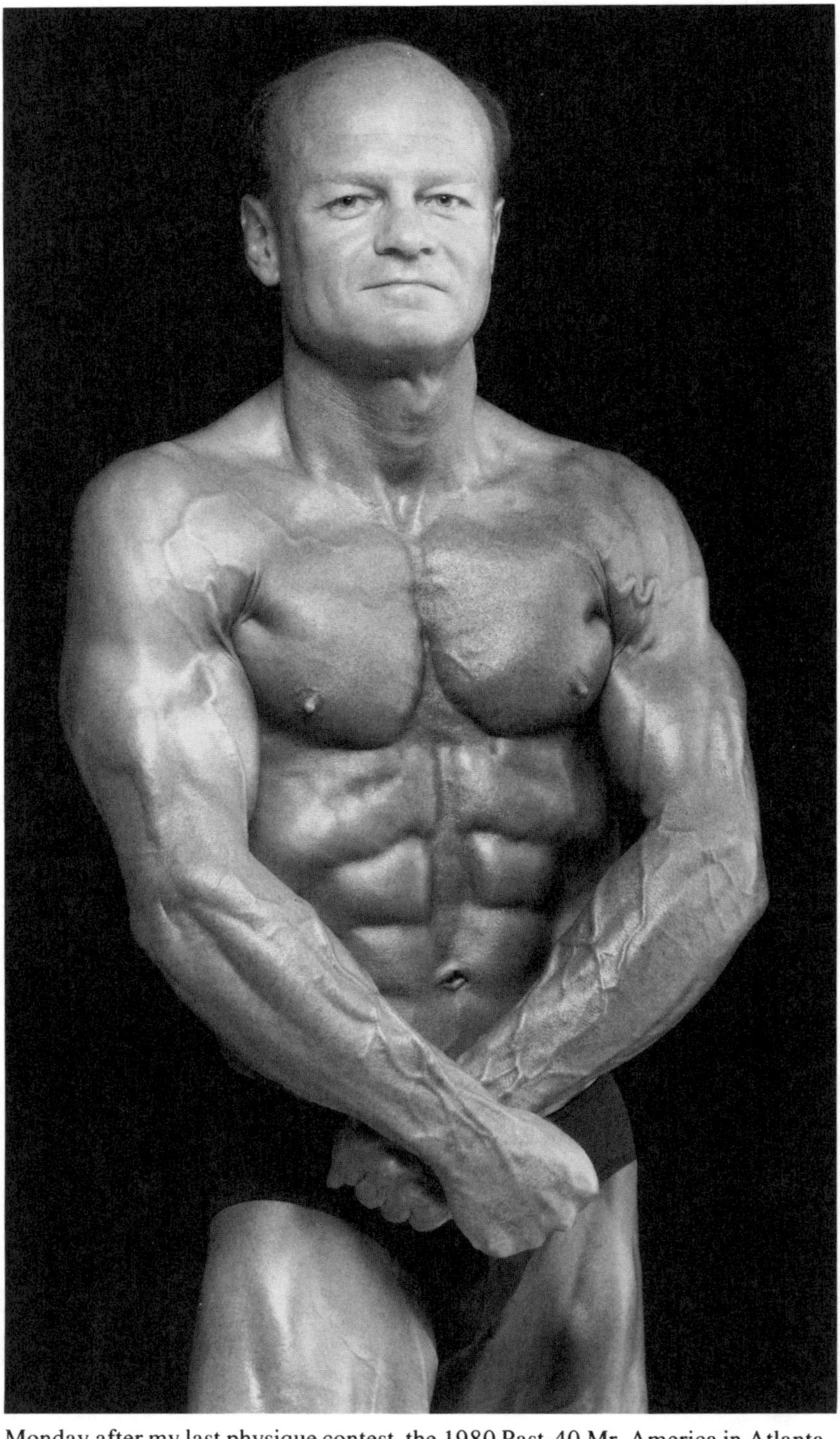

Monday after my last physique contest, the 1980 Past-40 Mr. America in Atlanta, where I placed 2nd in the middleweight class. *Photo by Bob Gardner.*

PHYSIOLOGICAL FACTORS 7

HEART RATE DECLINES?

Author's experience defies textbooks

You'd think it was written in stone: "Maximum heart rate (and thus cardiac output) slows every year after age 25." We all know that formula: 220 minus age. This equation, of course, assumes that the decline, one beat per year, is inescapable. That's what my exercise physiology textbook says: "This [decline] is progressive with advancing years and appears to occur to the same extent in both active and sedentary men and women."

Participants in a round-table discussion on training the older athlete in the *National Strength & Conditioning Association Journal* agreed. Vicky Foster, Ph.D., an assistant professor in the department of exercise and sports science at Colorado State University in Fort Collins, expressed what appeared to be the consensus of the group: "Although the standard deviation is broad, this formula [220 minus age] holds remarkably well for individuals of all fitness levels." Scott Going, Ph.D., an assistant research scientist in the exercise and sports science department at the University of Arizona, was even more emphatic: "The decline in maximal heart rate as a person ages is not altered by training."

Four Tests

Like everyone else, I accepted this apparently well-documented age-effect — that is, until recently. Now I'm not so sure. Here's why.

In 1977, when I was a few months short of 40, Lovelace Foundation for Medical Education and Research gave me my first maximal exercise stress test. My maximum heart rate was measured at 180, exactly in accord with the standard formula (220 minus 40 equals 180).

I was tested again just before my 44th birthday. Dr. Jack Leoppky, an associate scientist at Lovelace, conducted the test. He cautioned me that a loss of aerobic capacity is expected during the four-year time span between the two tests. It didn't happen, however. My aerobic capacity (VO_2 max) actually improved. And my maximum heart rate was 183, seven beats faster than the formula predicted (220 minus 44 equals 176).

In 1984 I was tested a third time, at the University of New Mexico Human Performance Laboratory. Between 1981 and 1984, my maximum oxygen consumption increased from 50 milliliters per minute per kilogram of bodyweight to 54. This time my maximal heart rate was 177, six beats slower than the last test, but still four beats faster than the formula predicted (220 minus 47 equals 173).

Serious Doubts

After three tests, the heart rate formula and my measured maximum seemed pretty much in line. But after my fourth test, at the Cooper Clinic when I was about to turn 51, I began to have serious doubts whether heart rate and aging are, in fact, inextricably bound.

In 1988, the Cooper Clinic measured my maximum heart rate at 183! More than a decade had passed since the first test, and my maximal heart rate was actually three beats faster. And 14 beats faster than predicted (220 minus 51 equals 169).

Now, I think it's fair to say that the standard formula and I have parted company. From age 40 to 51, the formula said my maximum heart rate would decline substantially. But it didn't. It remained essentially unchanged at about 180 beats per minute (the average of my four tests is 181).

I believe the truth is that researchers haven't studied enough men and women who, like me and many readers of this magazine, continue to train hard as they age. The jury is still out on the effect of exercise on maximum heart rate and other "well-documented" effects of aging.

Stay tuned, and keep training. We'll learn together.

NOTE:

In November, 1992, after I turned 55, the Cooper Clinic measured my maximum heart rate for a fifth time. This time it was 190 beats per minute, seven more than previously recorded and a full 25 beats faster than predicted! In my case, at least, the jury is in. The decline in maximum heart rate as a person ages can *be altered by training.*

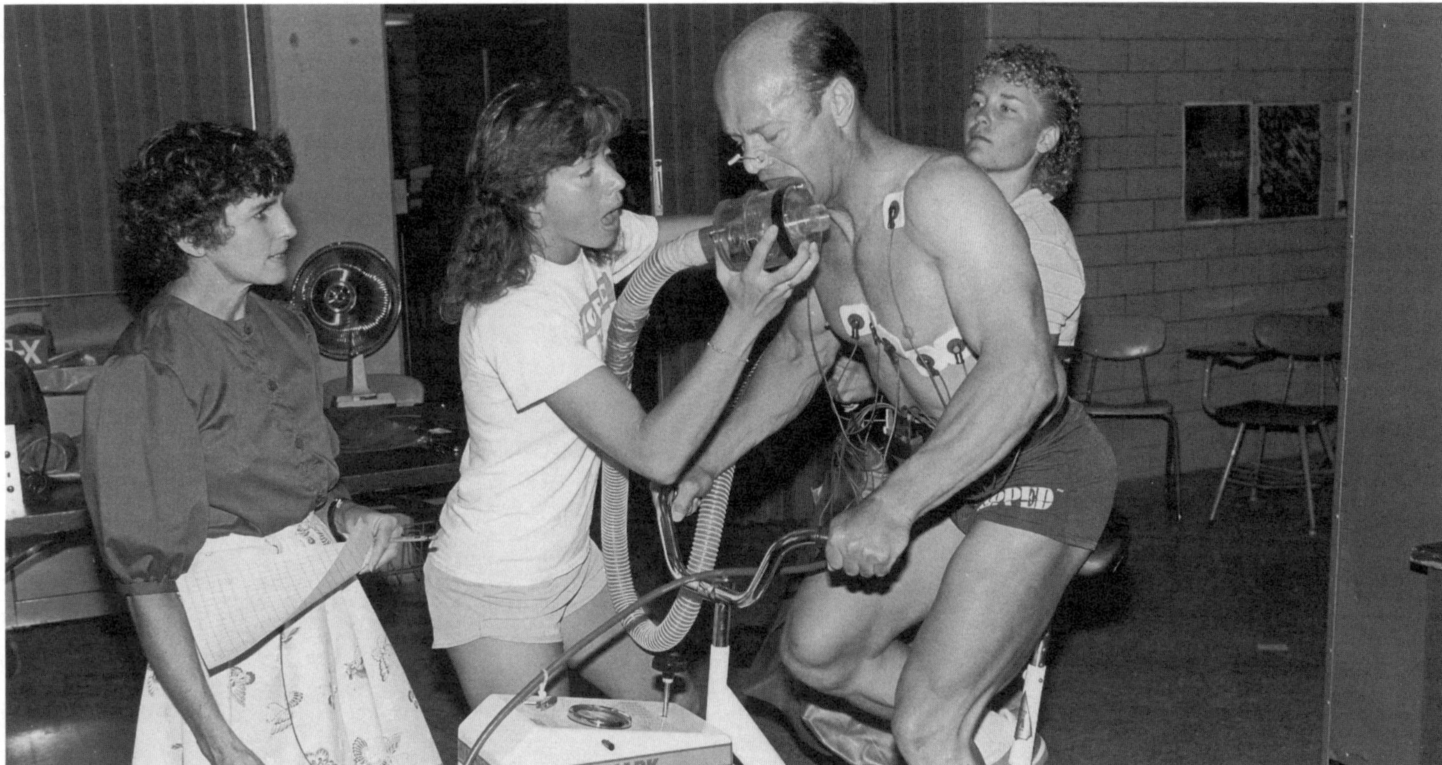

University of New Mexico Human Performance Laboratory, 1984, during my third maximum stress test. That's doctoral candidate Kay Steffens on the left. *Photo by Guy Appelman.*

THE METABOLISM MYTH

Your metabolism won't slow down if you don't

Q: *Avid readers of your column, my wife and I consider you an inspiration, especially since with my 50th birthday around the corner we have optimism that something can be done about the body composition shift. Pictures of people like yourself provide tangible, visible encouragement for the lean animal (hopefully) within all of us. I do have a concern, however. I've heard that as we get older the metabolic fires burn ever slower. Is that true? Will an aging metabolism work against my efforts to get lean and mean?*

A: Stop worrying. What you have heard is a myth. The metabolism does not slow down as you get older. Still, as you suggest, people do tend to gain fat as they get older. That's not because their metabolism has slowed, however. It's because they have lost muscle as a result of inactivity. The muscle that remains is as metabolically active as ever.

Metabolism Facts

Here are the facts as presented by Lawrence E. Lamb, MD, in his book *The Weighting Game* (Lyle Stuart, 1988). Researchers led by Dr. Ancel Keys at the University of Minnesota measured the energy requirements of people of different ages with different amounts of bodyfat. They found that the energy requirement of fat-free bodyweight (weight of the body minus the bodyfat) were remarkably constant for both men and women between the ages of 20 and 60. All the subjects, no matter what their sex or age, burned about 1.28 calories per hour per kilogram (2.2 pounds) of fat-free bodyweight, under basal conditions.

To really understand what's going on here, let's back up and take a hard look at this subject. What is metabolism, anyway? What can we do to speed up our metabolic furnaces to help us become lean and stay that way?

The dictionary tells us that metabolism is the chemical and physical processes continually going on in living organisms and cells, with the release of energy for all vital functions. In simpler terms, it's what happens as the body processes the food we eat. Two basic actions are involved. One is the breakdown phase (catabolism). This is when food is broken down and we lose weight. The other action is the building phase, which is called anabolism. This is when food is processed to form enzymes or other important chemicals, or new tissue, including muscle and fat. Both the catabolic and anabolic phases require energy.

You mentioned "metabolic fires." In this regard it's interesting to note that the anabolic process, the building phase, does not use oxygen or generate heat. The catabolic process, however, uses oxygen to burn

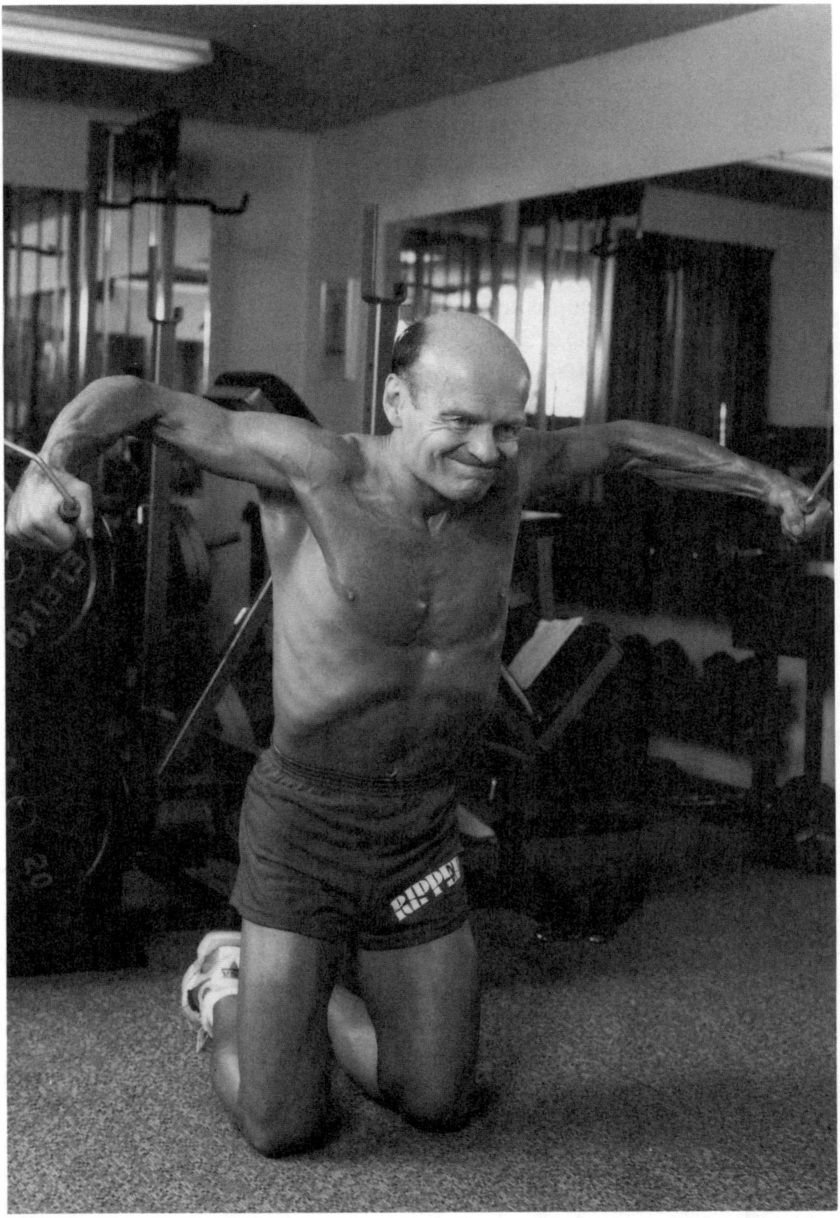

Photo by Pat Berrett.

food or tissue and does release heat. This means, of course, that heat is generated when you catabolize fat and lose weight. That's why you get hot and sweaty when you exercise. You're oxidizing (burning) calories and generating heat. On the other hand, no heat is involved when the body hooks amino acids together to form muscle, or goes through the process of storing excess calories as fat.

This brings us to the calorie balance equation, which is part and parcel of the metabolic process. It's what determines whether you gain or lose fat. Lamb, in his book, states the equation like this:

Calories in - calories used = calories deposited as fat + calories used in growth.

Age Doesn't Matter

Simply put, the calories in the food you eat that are not burned or used in growth are deposited as fat. You knew that, of course. Everybody knows that. The tricky part is manipulating the elements of the metabolic equation to lose fat and keep it off. It works the same no matter what your age. Let's see what can be done to reverse your body composition shift.

First, let's look at calories in. It's only common sense that if you reduce the calories you eat to a level below the calories you use, you'll lose weight. That's generally true, but there's a catch. If you cut calories too much, your body starts shutting the metabolic system down. It goes into a survival mode. Everything slows down. Your body conserves calories to get you through the crisis it perceives. Even the growth of your hair and fingernails slows. Unfortunately, the longer you stay on a calorie-restricted diet, the less effective it is in causing you to lose fat.

That's not to say you shouldn't watch what you eat. You should. As I explain in detail in my books, you should avoid calorie-dense foods and emphasize foods high in fiber and bulk. Eat plenty of fruit, vegetables and whole grains.

Turn On Your Furnace

The best results come from concentrating on the "calories used" side of the metabolic equation. This means exercise. Listen to Lamb: "Exercise literally turns on your metabolic furnace and liberates calories of heat. Dieting shuts down your metabolic furnace and causes you to use less calories."

Exercise burns calories while you exercise, and after exercise you continue to use more calories than at rest. Even mild exercise leaves you burning extra calories an hour later. If you exercise harder and longer, after 12 hours your energy requirements will still be elevated. And even at rest, your metabolically active muscles still use energy. The more muscle you have, the more calories you use, around the clock. That's why weight training is so important. It builds and maintains the calorie-burning muscle tissue that makes you lean. It keeps your metabolic fires burning strongly.

And don't let anyone tell you that you can't increase your muscle size and strength as you get older. As Lamb says in his book: "Developing an old muscle is just like developing a young muscle. You may need to be more careful and progress slower, but you can do it." Plus, keep training and pushing to your limit occasionally, and you'll keep your muscles.

Just remember this: Your metabolism won't slow down if you don't.

(For many more details, I urge you to read *The Weighting Game*. It's available from Ripped Enterprises.)

WHAT'S BROWN FAT?

Microscopic cells stablize body temperature and body weight

Q: *I see brown fat mentioned in news reports and articles from time to time. It has something to do with weight control, but that's about all I know. Can brown fat help me become leaner?*

A: In the last few years brown fat has received more press. That's because its existence in humans has been demonstrated only recently. It has long been known to exist in lower animals, where it serves two main functions. It helps them stay warm in cold weather, and it helps keep their bodyweight on an even keel when they overeat.

Most fat is white or yellow, but there are very small clusters of fat cells that are brown. These brown fat cells can be seen only under a microscope. Brown fat is scattered throughout the body, but most of it is located in the chest area and around the heart. The brown color is caused by a rich supply of capillaries and nerve endings.

These are a special kind of fat cells. They work like little furnaces, burning a lot of calories and fat, producing heat. That's quite different from ordinary yellow fat cells, which are passive, serving mainly as a place to store fat.

Animal Studies

Most of what is known about brown fat comes from animal studies. That's to be expected because animals can be dissected and their brown fat measured; in humans scientists have to infer the presence of brown fat from hot spots on the skin and changes in metabolism. There seems to be little doubt, however, that we do have significant amounts of brown fat; it's abundant in newborn infants, and its characteristics have been noted at all ages.

Two factors seem to stimulate brown fat action: cold and overeating. As noted, brown fat helps to stabilize an animal's temperature and bodyweight. As you might guess, brown fat is plentiful in animals that live in cold climates. Also, brown fat goes into action when animals eat too much. It burns the extra calories to heat the body rather than storing them in fat cells. This helps animals maintain the same weight. You can see why this would be helpful to an animal in the wild with an adequate but irregular food supply. A fat animal, after all, would be less able to find — or catch — its next meal.

Now, let's get to the real question: Can we enlist brown fat to keep us lean like wild animals? That's still an open question, but there's some evidence that we can. In his book *The Weighting Game* (Lyle Stuart, 1989), *Muscle & Fitness* columnist Lawrence E. Lamb, MD, cites the observation that brown fat develops around the neck of outdoor workers in Finland. This is consistent with animal studies and suggests that exposure to cold may activate or develop our brown fat cells. So for starters you may want to participate in outdoor activities during cold weather. That's not the main reason I walk outdoors year round, but it's one more thing to push me out the door when it's cold.

Brown Fat & Exercise

Probably the most encouraging word about brown fat, however, comes from fat-loss guru Covert Bailey. In his book *The Fit or Fat Woman* (Houghton Mifflin, 1989) Bailey says that brown fat seems to be associated with exercise. "Athletes have a more responsive brown fat mechanism, and as people become more athletic, the mechanism improves," he writes. Researchers have found, according to Bailey, that athletic people can pig out occasionally, consuming 2,000-3,000 excess calories, with no increase in bodyfat. Their brown fat comes to the rescue, "wasting" the extra calories so that they are released as heat rather than stored. Unfortunately, this doesn't seem to work for out-of-shape people, Bailey reports.

I've noticed this in my own case. For example, Easter Sunday my wife Carol and I enjoyed a big dinner with her family. I ate all I could hold, including three or four desserts. I have no idea how many calories I consumed, but, believe me, I overshot my calorie requirement by a bunch.

Monday morning my weight was up only three-quarters of a pound, and by midweek it was back to normal. I made no attempt to compensate by eating less early in the week. Still, I didn't gain an ounce. It was as if my Easter binge never happened. Was that my brown fat cells in action?

I doubt that anyone knows for sure. The jury is still out on the action of brown fat in humans. Covert Bailey says it's too early to give advice. He knows what he's going to do, however: "I am going to try to stimulate my brown fat in every way I can. I will exercise a lot and expose myself to outdoor cold."

That sounds sensible. Research takes a long time. It might be years before the results are in on brown fat. Like Bailey, I don't plan to wait.

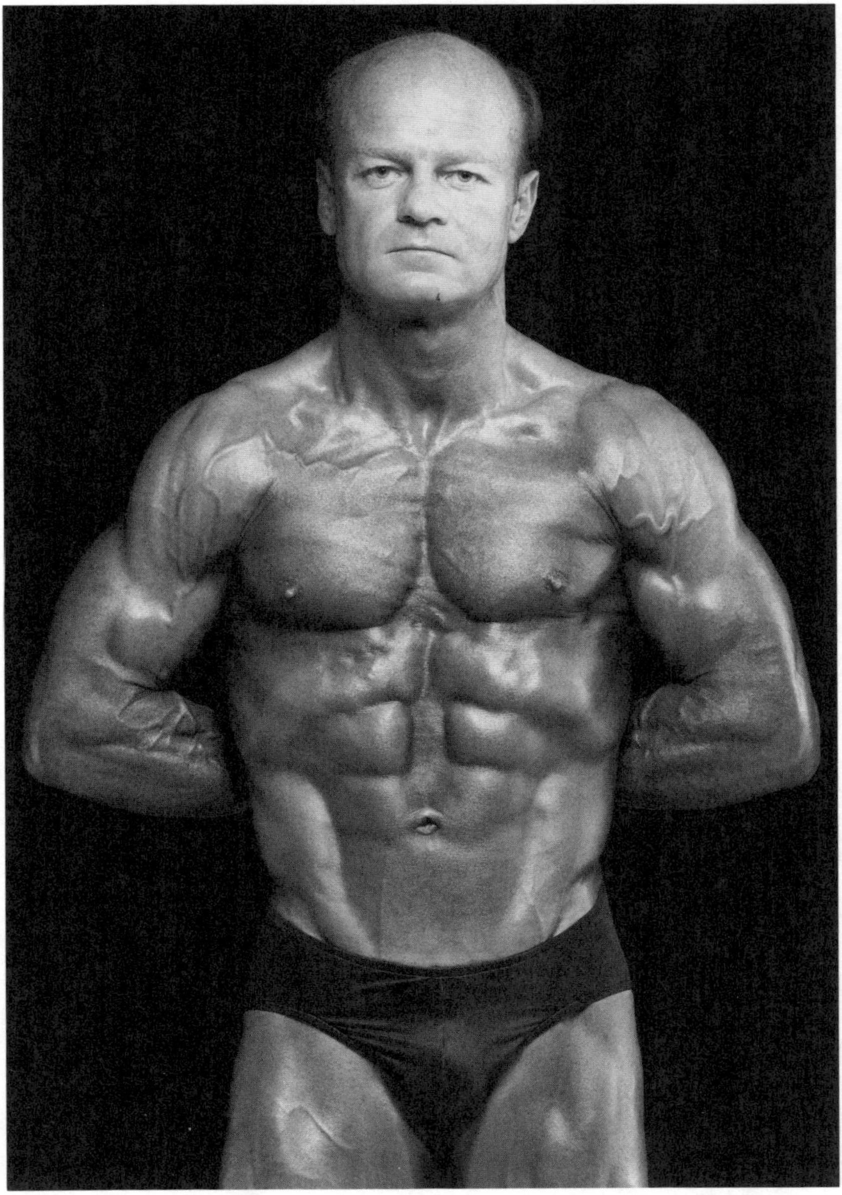

Photo by Bob Gardner.

As I see it, brown fat action is just one more in a long list of reasons to pursue our bodybuilding lifestyle.

THE FAT CELL FACTOR

Adult weight influenced by early fat cell development

Q: *I lost 70 pounds about four years ago. I've kept it off, but I still have a lot of body fat, especially around the stomach area.*

As a small boy I was always very chubby. I was very fat until the age of 14, when I started losing weight. I'm now 18.

I've been working out with weights off and on for about a year and also have been jogging and bike riding. I would be a much happier person if I could lose this fat around my stomach area. My mother says I should do more sit-ups.

A: First, congratulations on maintaining your big weight loss. You've already beaten the odds. The photo enclosed shows you're now of normal bodyweight. Most people regain the weight they lose in a short time. Your success to date — and your obvious determination — suggest that further improvement lies ahead. Success breeds success.

Spot Reducing

Fat biopsies show it doesn't work

I'm sure your mother means well, but she is misinformed about sit-ups. Exercise physiologists will tell you that spot reducing doesn't work. Fat biopsies taken from the abdominal region, upper back, and buttocks of subjects who performed sit-ups every day for 27 days showed that the fat cells in the exercised abdominal region did not become smaller than those in the unexercised buttock and upper back regions.

The fat over your stomach belongs to your whole body. The only way to reduce the size of the fat cells in one area is to reduce them over the entire body. Sit-ups should be a part of your training program, but exercise for the large muscles of the body (and diet) is the key to fat reduction. Weight training, jogging and biking is the right approach.

Fat Cells

Obese adults have more

Now, I have both good and bad news. *Exercise Physiology,* the excellent text by Drs. William D. McArdle, Frank I. Katch and Victor L. Katch (Lea & Febiger, 3rd Edition, 1991), explains that fat cell development is a key factor in weight control. The fact that you were very overweight as a child suggests that you have a large number of fat cells. This makes body fat reduction more difficult. The good part is that your adolescent weight reduction curtailed fat cell development at a critical stage.

Before adulthood, body fat increases in two ways: by enlargement of individual fat cells and by an increase in the total number of fat cells. The number of fat cells becomes stable sometime before adulthood; any weight gain or loss after that is usually related to a change in the size of the individual cells.

Obese adults typically have many more fat cells than normal individuals. According to *Exercise Physiology*, a non-obese person has approximately 25 to 30 billion fat cells, whereas the number of fat cells in the "extremely obese" may be as high as 260 billion. When an adult loses weight, there is a decrease in fat cell size but no change in cell number. So, for an obese adult to reach normal weight individual fat cells must shrink and actually become smaller in size than the fat cells of non-obese individuals. In one study where 19 obese adults reduced their body mass by more than 150 pounds, their fat cell size shrunk to about one-third the size of the fat cells of normal, non-obese subjects. As you might expect, this makes it more difficult for them to maintain their loss.

A bummer, huh? Don't be discouraged. Those are extreme cases. Your situation is much more hopeful.

Good News

Childhood fat loss helps later

Increases in the number of fat cells appear to involve three critical periods: the last trimester of pregnancy, the first year of life and the adolescent growth spurt prior to adulthood. You apparently developed greater than the normal number of fat cells early in life. That's the bad news. The good news is that your big weight reduction came early in adolescence when significant fat cell increases often occur. You took the bull by the horns at just the right time. Your weight reduction at age 14, no doubt, prevented the development of additional fat cells which would have made things more difficult for you in later years. You should experience very little further increase in fat cell number. You probably have only a few more fat cells than normal. Your job now is to reduce the size of those cells.

Build Muscle

Pumping iron makes you lean

As mentioned earlier, you're already on the right track. Like you, I started serious weight training in my early teens. That launched me on a lifetime of leanness. Weight training is very important to fat reduction, because it builds and maintains muscle tissue, thereby keeping your calorie-burn level up high. I suggest that you build as much muscle as you can. This magazine and my book *Ripped 2* will help you achieve that goal.

I didn't take up aerobic exercise until I was about 30, so you have a head start on me there. By all means, continue. Endurance exercise not only burns calories while you exercise and for a time thereafter, it also switches your body chemistry to a fat-burning mode; it alters your metabolism in a way that naturally produces a leaner body. For details on aerobics as a fat-loss adjunct to bodybuilding, read *Ripped 3.*

Diet, of course, should continue to be a major part of your fat loss plan. A fat-loss diet should create a *slight* calorie deficit to burn off excess fat stores. At the same time — and this is important — a properly designed diet must provide enough calories to make you feel full and satisfied. If you feel hungry and deprived, you're not eating enough. You're probably eating the wrong kind of food as well. My books will help you there, too.

You should be very encouraged — and proud — that you have lost a great deal of weight and kept it off for more than four years. Regularity and further refinement of your diet and exercise program will get rid of the flab that remains around your middle. Just keep doing what you're doing, but do it smarter. You'll be amazed how much your fat cells will shrink.

CHAPTER EIGHT

PSYCHOLOGICAL FACTORS

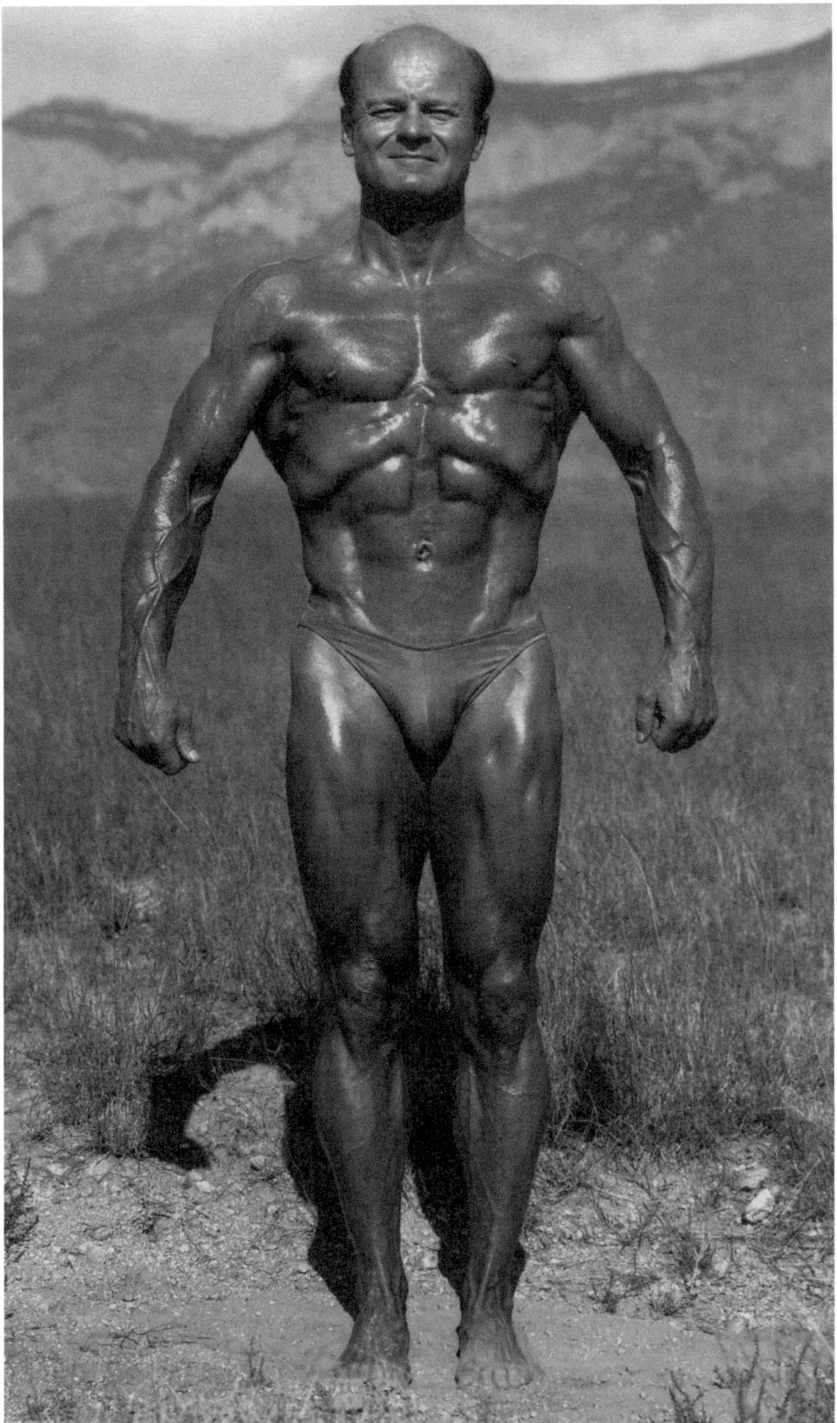

Photo by Guy Appelman.

PSYCHOLOGICAL FACTORS 8

THE STRESS FIGHTER

Exercise, both aerobic and anaerobic, works for almost everyone

We all feel stressed out from time to time. Our problems exceed our resources for coping with them, and we feel stressed. I know I sometimes feel overwhelmed trying to keep up with everything: training, law practice, mail-order business, correspondence, investments, writing deadlines, family matters, and on and on. I remember I especially felt overburdened during and after my father's final illness. In addition to the emotional pain of losing my dad, management of the family affairs fell to me as well. I felt like a juggler with too many balls in the air. Nevertheless, it didn't take me long to regain my equilibrium and feel on top of things again. Fortunately, I seem to cope with stress pretty well.

Dr. Raymond B. Flannery, Jr., a psychologist at Harvard Medical School and a member of the Department of Psychiatry at Cambridge Hospital, Cambridge, Massachusetts, has made a study of people who respond to demanding situations without losing their sense of well-being. I've always been interested in how people cope with stress, and the experience of losing my father has made me all the more interested in Flannery's findings, which were set out in the February 1989 *Harvard Medical School Health Letter.* I was fascinated — and more than a little reassured — to learn the characteristics of people who cope effectively. I believe *Muscle & Fitness* readers will be interested as well.

Flannery says the coping strategies of the stress-resistant person fall into four main categories. Because of space limitations, I'll just touch on three of Flannery's categories, and then I'll elaborate on the fourth stress fighter because it's of special interest to *M&F* readers. It is, of course, exercise.

Stress & Exercise

First, stress-resistant people tend to maintain reasonable personal control in their lives. On the other hand, people who succumb to stress are more likely to approach problems passively. As an example, I took control of my father's affairs, determined what needed to be done, and then put things in order one by one. I didn't passively turn the job over to others.

Secondly, stress-resistant people are personally committed to a goal of some kind. This enhances their sense of meaningful participation in life. Stress-prone people are more likely to indicate they are bored and unable to find something that interests them.

Thirdly, people who cope well tend to be actively engaged with other people. A stressed person is more likely to be socially isolated.

Finally, the stress-resistant person usually takes charge of his or her self physically. About 80% of the stress-resistant people Flannery studied engaged in regular exercise, compared to 20% of the stress prone.

Stone-Age Heritage

Interpreting his findings, Flannery commented, "The hallmarks of contemporary urban life are that it is both sedentary and fast-paced." This, he says, may be incompatible with the physiology we inherited from our stone-age ancestors. Flannery speculates that the stress-resistant person lives more like the hunters and gatherers "who represent the experience of humanity until very recent times. . . ." One thing is sure. The hunters and gatherers from which we evolved were active; they had to walk, run and work hard physically just to survive.

The Physician and Sportsmedicine (June 1988) reviewed the scientific literature to see what we actually know about exercise and stress reduction. The search revealed that we don't have all the answers, but we do know that many people exercise to feel better psychologically as well as physically. And it seems to work. Here's a few of the facts we know or have reason to believe:

- A number of studies show that exercise and fitness reduce the intensity of the stress response; they reduce the increases in blood pressure and heart rate associated with stress. They also shorten the time it takes a person to recover from stress.
- The effect of exercise on stress seems to vary with the type of exercise. According to Peter Seraganian, Ph.D., aerobic fitness "promotes rapid recovery from an emotional experience." Seraganian, an associate professor of psychology at Concordia University in Montreal, and his associates studied the relationship between fitness level and the reaction to stress in 45 men between the ages of 20-50.

The researchers measured heart rate and electrodermal activity to assess reaction to laboratory-induced stress. Here are the results:

• The aerobically fit men in the group recovered faster after exposure to stress than the unfit men. The unfit group members didn't react more strongly to the stressors than the fit men, but they felt the effects longer. "This is an important point," says Seraganian, "because a sluggish recovery extends the period of time during which a person may be more vulnerable to a hyper reaction."

In support of this finding, Robert Cantu, MD, chief of the Neurosurgery Service and director of the Service of Sports Medicine at Emerson Hospital in Concord, Massachusetts, points out that aerobic fitness often is associated with lowered heart rate and blood pressure. Stress, of course, causes heart rate and blood pressure to rise. Cantu believes that the effects of stress are bound to be less apparent in a fit person, who has lower blood pressure and heart rate to begin with. He also points out that aerobic training reduces the level of the fight-or-flight hormones, further reducing the end results of stress.

Resistance Training

As is so often the case, most of the research on exercise and stress involves aerobic exercise. What about anaerobic exercise such as weight training? Some argue that anaerobic exercise does not create the physiological changes that are linked to stress reduction. They say that weight training might even be counterproductive since it raises blood pressure. On the contrary, however, research suggests that anaerobic exercise, like aerobic exercise, does reduce stress.

Debra J. Crews, MS, a doctoral candidate in exercise science at Arizona State University in Tempe, told the American College of Sports Medicine that her research suggests that anaerobic exercise reduces the stress response as effectively as aerobic training. According to Crews, anaerobic exercise, such as weight training on machines, should reduce physiological responses during stress, "since that is what anaerobic activity is about — you stress and recover, stress and recover."

What's more, in one area of stress reduction, weight training may have a leg up on any other form of exercise. "It isn't the amount of stress that is important; it is what amount you perceive to be there," says Larry Tucker, Ph.D., associate professor of health promotion at Auburn University in Alabama.

Probably more than any other form of exercise, weight training produces a strong, lean, good-looking body that is almost guaranteed to enhance self-esteem and self-image. People who feel good about themselves as a result of weight training are inclined to perceive negative factors as less stressful than an unfit person with a poor self-image.

Finally, the act of exercise itself may help reduce stress. John Howard, Ph.D., a professor of business administration at the University of Western Ontario School of Business in London, Ontario, reminds us,

"One of the undervalued effects of exercise is the draining off of excess energy." In short, it's hard to feel stressed when you're pooped from a workout. "Following a workout, a fit individual usually experiences an afterglow," adds Howard.

Admittedly, we don't know everything there is to know about exercise as a stress fighter. Nevertheless, in my book, Howard got it right when he told *The Physician and Sportsmedicine:* "Exercise probably works for almost everybody. I've never seen it fail."

A WINNING EXPERIENCE

How I beat the most important competitor of all, myself

I didn't win — didn't even come close — but I was a winner nonetheless.

Indoor rowing competition, which simulates rowing on the water, using a machine made by Concept II, Inc., is an ideal second sport for bodybuilders. It requires power — especially in the legs and back —and endurance, qualities that must be possessed in abundance by the modern-day bodybuilder. This is especially true now that bodybuilders use aerobic exercise to become lean and defined, to get ripped.

As a former Olympic lifter, I found the rowing motion similar to the Barbell Clean, where the weight is lifted from the floor to shoulder level in one motion. On the Concept II rower you start pushing with your legs and hips, the strongest muscles in the body, then your lower back muscles, the next strongest, kick in, and finally you end up pulling with your lats, traps and arms. It's a long and smooth but powerful movement. It feels good; there's no undue stress on the joints. You couldn't prove it by me, but they say it's just like real rowing.

Indoor Rowing Races

I've been rowing on the Concept II for about two years. I had read that indoor rowing competitions using this machine are held in the United States and Europe. The competition angle is part of what attracted me to the Concept II rowing machine.

After purchasing my unit, I learned that Concept II compiles a world ranking each year, an ordered list of personal bests for 2,500 meters rowed on their machine. Times are grouped in 10-year age classses for both women and men. There's no official distinction for weight classes, but the ranking denotes men and women weighing over and under 165 and 135 pounds, respectively. The best times are generally by the heavier rowers. For example, the world record is held by Matthias Siejkowski, a 6′10″ 250-pound Olympic rowing gold medalist from

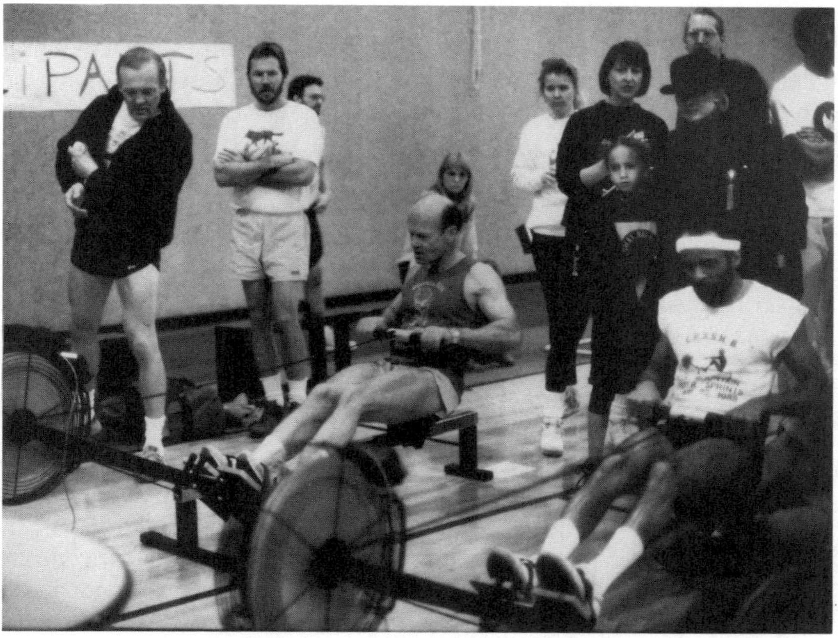

Fellow "oarsman" cheers me on at the Rocky Mountain Rowing Club competition in Denver. *Photo by Carol Bass.*

West Germany. As I already suggested, rowing is a strength athlete's sport.

I practiced for a while and then sent my best time to Concept II. The 1989 world ranking included about 5,800 men and women from all over the world. I placed 66th out of 154 men in the 50-59 age category. Among those weighing less than 165 pounds I was 11th.

A Challenge

I had just begun casual and not-too-enthusiastic training for the 1990 world ranking when an entry form came in the mail from the Rocky Mountain Rowing Club for a competition to be held in Denver. I said to myself: "This is it! Competition is just what the doctor ordered!"

At Denver's Cherry Creek Athletic Club, where the competition was held, rowing machines were set up eight abreast across the gym floor. Each machine was connected to a big television screen placed in front of the rowers. A crowd of rooters stood behind the "oarsmen."

Dropping the flag, the starter yelled, "Row!"

The "sculls" moved electronically across the screen, the announcer calling out the names of the leaders and those in neck-and-neck battles, as the crowd cheered us on.

Like any all-out effort, rowing 2,500 meters [a little over 1½ miles] is tough. It's like doing Deadlifts nonstop for about 10 minutes. To do your best you really need a kick in the pants of some sort. As George Sheehan has written, "Competition is simply each of us seeking our absolute best with the help of each other."

Personal Best

As I had hoped, the rowing competition motivated me to train hard and did indeed push me to a new personal best record. As stated at the outset, I did not win the rowing competition. In the heats I made a personal record for 2,500 meters and qualified for the finals in the veterans category, where I placed seventh. The winner in my age group did 9:03.0. He and a number of other competitors showed me what is possible and convinced me that I can do much better.

Still, as good as the men were, the performance that impressed me the most was by a young woman. I'm guessing she weighed a little less than me. I don't remember her exact time, but it was under 9:30. She rowed with powerful strokes, long and even. She was terrific! More than anything else, seeing her performance convinced me that I was setting my sights too low, that I am capable of a much better rowing time.

I focus on this woman's performance because, as I've said, weight and height have a lot to do with rowing ability. Almost all the best times are by big, tall people. That was true of the top over-50 rower in Denver; he outweighed me by about 50 pounds and was at least 6 inches taller. That's why the woman's performance was so outstanding. She had no height or weight advantage and still beat my time by a substantial margin.

Breaking Through

It's like the four-minute mile barrier. Once Roger Bannister broke through, the floodgates opened. Runners all over the world came to believe they could run a four-minute mile, and they did. The woman rower did the same thing for me.

In my first rowing session upon returning home I hit a level of performance that I would have considered over my head only a few days earlier. With the woman rower as my inspiration, I'm going to spend a few weeks adjusting to a faster pace, and then I'm convinced that I will establish a new personal record and maybe even move up on the Concept II world list for 1990.

So I was a winner after all. I did a personal best and came away inspired to do even better next time. I found a new mountain that I can realistically expect to climb. I beat the most important competitor of all, myself.

NEVER MAKE IT EASY

"We are unhappy, not because of things we lack but because we have potentials that have not been realized."
— George Sheehan, M.D.

My psychologist friend Richard Winett was amazed that I would enter the indoor rowing competition described here last month. After all, he observed, I'm not an aerobics specialist, and I'd be up against some awesome rowers. Why put my reputation on the line? Well, I almost didn't enter, but it wasn't because of the competition or my reputation. The obstacle that stood in my way was a more personal demon. Let me tell you about it.

Last year, as I trained to make a personal record for inclusion in the Concept II Rowing Machines world ranking, I developed quite an aversion to the rower. I dreaded the pain and discomfort that is part and parcel of an all-out 2,500-meter row. "The event is comparable to running a 440-yard dash for two miles," a coach at the 1990 World Indoor Rowing Championships told *The Wall Street Journal.* "A normal body shouldn't be put under such strain," she added.

My personal agony, however, had a macabre tinge. During hard rowing sessions, as I fought to get my breath, I sometimes felt like I was suffocating, sort of a feeling of impending doom. In particular, when the performance monitor showed the next work interval fast approaching, I felt like I was trapped on a mechanical monster. Most unpleasant, to say the least. Still, the memory had faded with the passage of time, and I thought I could handle it, especially with a competition coming up in five weeks.

Impending Doom?

With so little time to prepare, I decided to simply do a 2,500-meter time trial every week, along with some interval work. I planned to increase the intensity for four weeks, taper off the last week and be ready to go for a personal record at the competition. That worked fine for the first two time trials; the first week was pretty comfortable, and I picked up the pace during the second week without any particular difficulty. During the third week, however, as I sped up more, the feeling of impending doom returned. In about the middle of the 2,500-meter piece I just didn't want to continue. I was right on pace, doing fine really, but the suffocating feeling came back. I just didn't want to face the last 1,000 meters. So I stopped.

I walked around for a few minutes, got myself together, and finished the workout strongly.

Later, I explained to my wife Carol what had happened. She listened patiently, as she always does, and suggested that maybe I should pass on the rowing meet. I seriously considered that option, but only for a few minutes. Then, as the Nike ad says, I decided to "just do it." As it turned out, that was the correct decision, but it was a little more complicated than the advertising slogan would suggest.

At this point, you're probably wondering why I would want to put myself through such unpleasantness. Basically because I knew I was capable of a new record row. As George Sheehan, MD, says in his wonderful book *Personal Best* (Rodale Press, 1989): "We are unhappy not because of things we lack but because we have potentials that have not been realized."

I've been competing and improving all my life. Why should I stop now, I asked myself. "The best way to play the aging game," Sheehan advises, "is to concede nothing. Never make it easy for yourself."

First Principle Of Fitness

Okay, I was going to compete. But how would I overcome my aversion to maximum effort on the rowing machine? It didn't take long to figure it out. I simply took the advice I've given many times: Make it fun. As Sheehan reminds us in *Personal Best,* "That has *always* been the first principle of fitness: What you do must be enjoyable, or you will

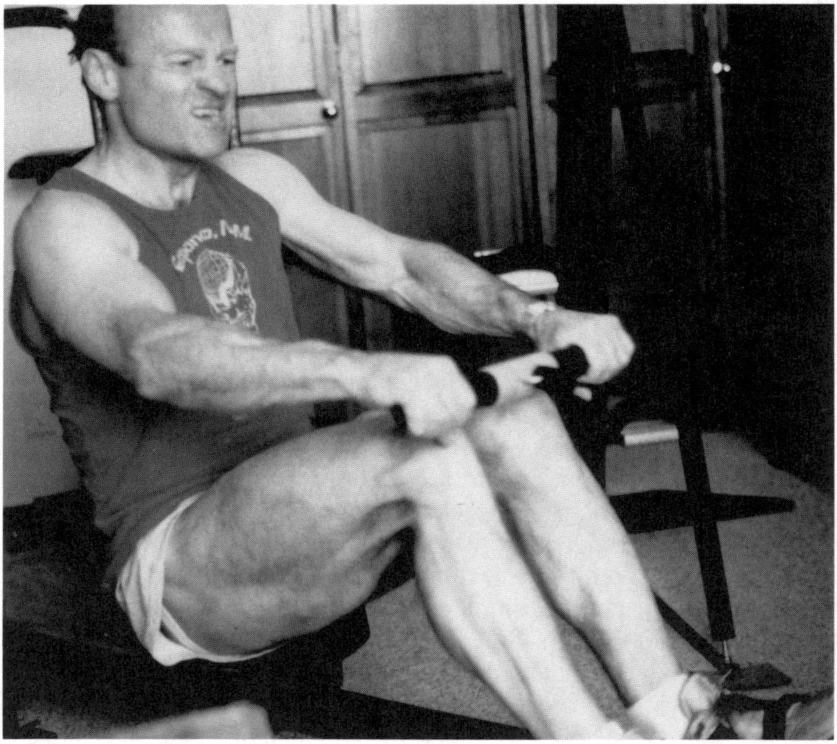

My 2500 meter PR row after returning home from Denver. *Photo by Carol Bass.*

not persist in it."

After the rowing session where the feeling of doom returned, I wrote in my training diary: "Stop doing 2,500 meters. Do other distances." Doing the competitive distance over and over put a monkey on my back. I had to keep topping myself workout after workout. After thinking about it, I knew I'd do better by varying the meters rowed, doing more than 2,500 meters some days, less on other days, and get the record through the back door. It worked. I did something different each workout leading up to the competition. In the process, I made personal records for everything from 20 minutes to one minute, with the exception of the approximately 10 minutes it takes to row the competitive distance. This prepared me nicely for 2,500 meters. And it was a lot more pleasant. Every session was a new ballgame, with no psychological baggage from the time before.

Forget To Breathe?

I made one other adjustment. After hearing about my problem, Guy Trucano, my overnight typist, left me a note with a very perceptive query: "Do you ever find that when you're concentrating on something, you forget to breathe?" After initially dismissing the idea, I decided he might be right. When rowing hard, as when lifting a heavy weight, the tendency is to hold your breath. I focused on regular breathing after that, and I believe it helped.

Finally, I suspect that subconsciously I associated my breathlessness on the rower with my father's trouble breathing when he was dying. I know that my perception of impending doom was not entirely physical, because I've experienced the same feeling just thinking about rowing. The recognition that my problem might have a psychological component helped.

Was all the effort and analysis worthwhile? You bet! As readers of last month's column already know, I made a new PR at the rowing competition, 9:46.1, and came away convinced I could do better still. I did. Three weeks later, I proudly sent Concept II a spanking new PR for their world list — 9:32.1.

Follow George Sheehan's advice (and mine): "Don't take things easy, take things hard." Because, as Dr. Sheehan says, "Becoming the best you can be makes you feel the best you can feel."

THE JOY OF GETTING LEAN

The "flow" formula for success

Q: *My goal is to get ripped to celebrate my next birthday. which is in seven months. At present I'm carrying about 15% bodyfat. I'd like your advice, please.*

A: The best advice I can give you — it will practically ensure your success — is: Enjoy the process. If you enjoy an activity, you're likely to persist in it. If you don't enjoy something, you'll probably quit.

In my book *The Lean Advantage,* I wrote: "I've found that I'm happiest when I'm working hard to achieve some goal. I enjoy the process of moving closer and closer to the goal of peak condition. The process of losing fat and gaining muscle, getting ripped, is gratifying in and of itself."

This is not a new idea. As Mihaly Csikszentmihalyi (let's just call him "Dr. C."), a professor and former chairman of the department of psychology at the University of Chicago, says in his new book *Flow: The Psychology of Optimal Experience* (Harper & Row, 1990), since the days of Aristotle it has been known that "Periods of struggling to overcome challenges are what people find to be the most enjoyable times of their lives."

"Flow" is the term Dr. C. uses to describe those times when people report feelings of enjoyment, concentration and deep involvement, or a genuinely enjoyable state of consciousness. Paraphrasing Dr. C., here's the blueprint followed by people who experience flow: They set appropriate goals, closely monitor feedback, and when they reach their goal, they up the ante, setting increasingly complex challenges for themselves. Let's explore Dr. C.'s formula for flow in the context of your situation.

Realistic Goal

Your idea of targeting your birthday seven months away to get ripped fits the flow formula perfectly. I've successfully used the target-date approach many times — a contest, a photo session, a trip to the Cooper Clinic, etc. Setting a goal charts your course and focuses your efforts. It's important, however, that your goal is realistic and achievable. Don't bite off more than you can chew. One pound of fat per week is the most you should try to lose. (As you approach maximum leanness the rate of reduction should be even less.) If you attempt to lose faster, you'll probably lose muscle, and you'll surely make yourself miserable. Believe me, starving yourself is not the way to get ripped — or experience flow.

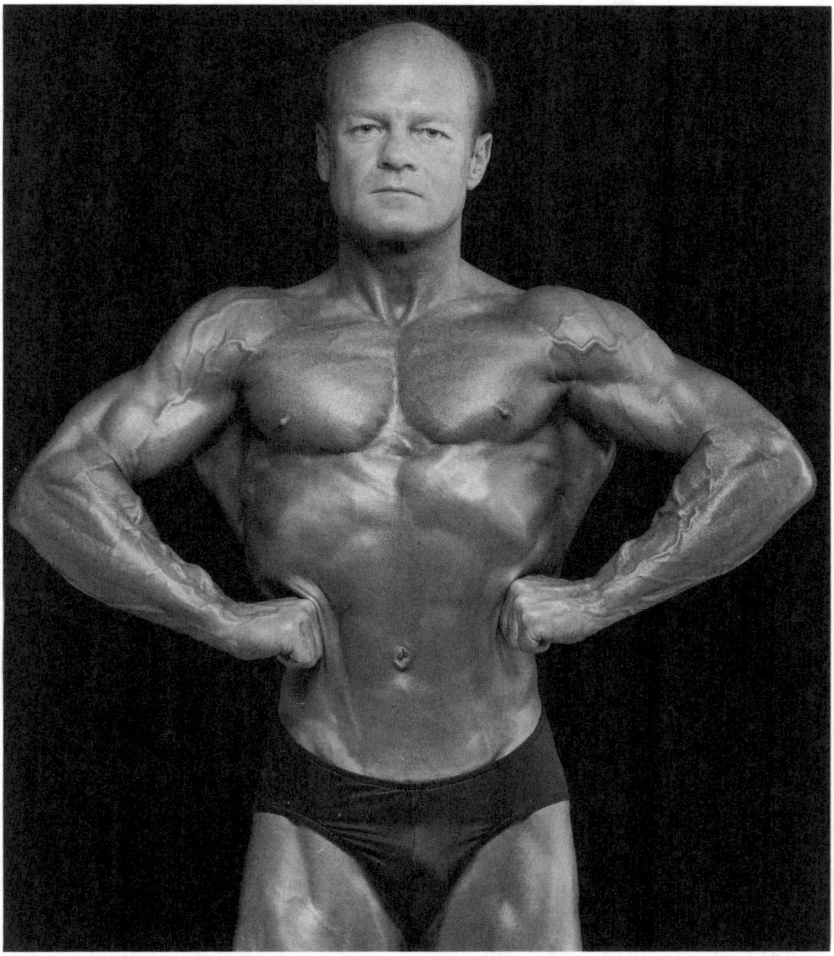

Photo by Bob Gardner.

Positive Feedback

Feedback will be critical to your success. Probably more than anything else, feedback showing that you're moving toward your goal, positive feedback, makes the fat loss process enjoyable. In short, success breeds success.

Losing 1 pound of fat (or less) each week is a clear-cut goal. That's good because it means you can measure your progress precisely. Your feedback will be clear and immediate, and that's extremely satisfying.

Follow the advice in my books and you'll have no trouble losing fat each week. Sure, you're bound to have some ups and downs — we all do — but the trend will be clear.

Monitor your progress by weighing yourself and measuring your waist each morning. I keep a record of these measurements by my bathroom scale. Here's an important tip: Week-to-week changes are more important than what happens day to day. That's because eating and activity tend to fall into weekly patterns. For example, most people eat more loosely on the weekends and, therefore, weigh more on Monday and Tuesday. For that reason, your weight on the same day of the previous week is usually more significant than whether you gained or lost from the day before. So focus on the weekly trend, not changes from one day to the next.

Monitor your waist measurement along with your bodyweight, because waistline reduction is a sure sign of fat loss.

Plus, if you have access to one of the new infrared bodyfat testers, I suggest that you use it as an additional source of feedback. Again, it's important to focus on weekly rather than daily changes.

Challenge

The final element of the flow formula is setting increasingly complex challenges for yourself. When you reach a goal, you must up the ante. A general principle, according to Dr. C., is that any activity can become enjoyable if you "take control of it, and cultivate it in the direction of greater complexity."

So don't allow your diet and training to get stuck in a rut. With a little study and imagination the process of getting ripped can be a never-ending challenge. Here are some suggestions.

- Don't settle for the tasteless and boring tuna and egg white diets. Learn about enjoyable, low-fat, high-fiber eating. You can start by studying the recipe plans and commentaries in *Ripped 3*.
- Don't settle for only one form of aerobic exercise. Train your whole body — arms and legs — with a variety of exercises. In addition to the usual jogging and biking, try rowing, climbing, skiing and stationary biking with push-pull arm action. Take advantage of the high-tech performance monitors available on many modern-day exercise machines; they can turn a humdrum exercise into an exciting challenge.
- Last but certainly not least, make your weight training progressive and varied. Challenge yourself to constantly lift heavier weights. Use high and low repetitions, and a variety of exercises. For ideas, Bill Pearl's book *Keys to the Inner Universe* describe every weight training exercise imaginable. And my book *Ripped 3* explains how different repetition ranges make lifting more productive — and fun.

I've been training most of my life, and I still find joy — and success — in the process. You can do the same. Just remember the components of flow: goals, feedback and challenge. Learn to enjoy the process of getting ripped and you'll be a winner every time.

LEARNED OPTIMISM

A "can do" attitude leads to success in bodybuilding — and life

Q: *My son Gary and I just finished rebuilding the engine on a 1985 Buick. I'd like to tell you about it because it relates to bodybuilding.*

We both have worked on engines before, but neither of us had tackled one of the new computer-controlled front-wheel-drive engines before. When we opened the hood, it looked like a plate of spaghetti — there were so many wires, hoses and assorted thingamajigs. Most people would have thought it was hopeless. But we piled right in.

It took us four days to assemble and install the new parts. The last hurdle was reprogramming the onboard computer.

The engine started right up. With a few adjustments we had it running like new.

What does this have to do with bodybuilding? Attitude. How many people would have said, "No way." Gary and I don't think that way, however. The truth is, we can do almost anything if we believe we can. This "can do" attitude is clearly evident in your column and throughout the pages of Muscle & Fitness. *That's why I'm so gung-ho about the bodybuilding lifestyle.*

A: You make a crucial point. In *Learned Optimism* (Alfred A. Knopf, 1991) Martin E.P. Seligman, Ph.D., one of the world's leading authorities on motivation, presents scientific evidence that optimists get along better than pessimists in almost every facet of life: at school, at work, in personal relationships and in sports. According to Seligman, optimists respond better to adversity of all kinds. What's more, they have better physical health and may even live longer. The key seems to be what we say to ourselves when we confront failure and disappointment, or a daunting task like rebuilding a car engine.

Pessimists, according to Seligman, respond with helplessness; they give up. Optimists, on the other hand, persevere. Like you and your son, they assess the situation, and they act constructively. Interestingly, our "explanatory style" — Seligman's term for the manner in which we explain setbacks to ourselves — affects our immune system; optimists have better immune activity than pessimists.

Most of us learn to be optimists or pessimists in childhood and adolescence, and then, for good or bad, we carry this basic attitude with us throughout life. Happily, a negative explanatory cycle can be changed to positive.

Bodybuilding & Attitude

I agree with you that bodybuilding can play an important part in shaping one's attitude. Let me tell you about the basic research done by

Seligman and his colleagues on learned helplessness or optimism, and then how weight training played a pivotal role in shaping my own way of looking at life.

In 1965, Seligman, while a graduate student in the department of experimental psychology at the University of Pennsylvania, performed the first experiment showing that animals can be taught helplessness. One group of dogs was given escapable shock. By pushing a panel with its nose, a dog in that group could turn off the shock. The dog had control because it could escape the shock. A second group of dogs was given exactly the same shocks as the first, but no response they made had any effect. They had no control; they couldn't escape. A third group was given no shocks at all.

Once the dogs went through the experiment, each was put in a large box with two compartments, separated by a low wall. In the first compartment they received a shock, but they could easily escape the

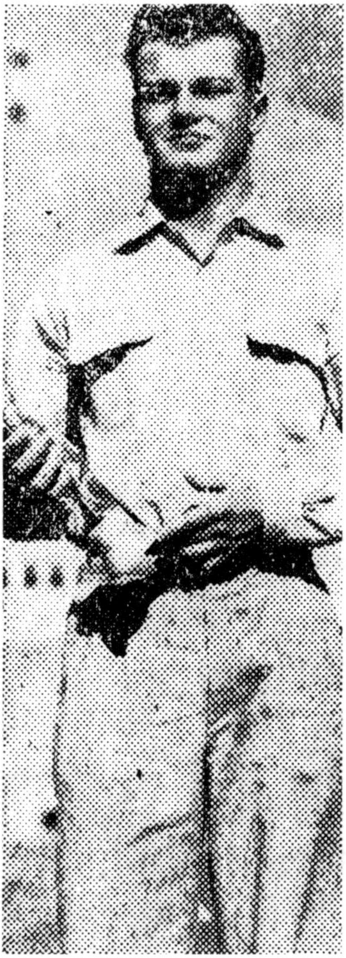

This fuzzy photo shows me on the victory stand after winning the state high school pentathlon championship. That early success taught me that perseverance pays and set the pattern for the rest of my life.

shock by jumping over the barrier into the other side of the box.

Within seconds the dogs that had been taught to control shocks discovered that they could jump over the barrier and escape. The dogs that earlier had received no shocks discovered the same thing, also in a matter of seconds. But the dogs who had found that nothing they did mattered made no effort to escape, even though they could easily see over the low barrier to the shockless zone of the box.

Those dogs just gave up and lay down, even though they were being regularly shocked by the box. They never found that they could easily escape. Those dogs had learned that they had no control, that they were helpless.

Learned Helplessness

It turns out that learned helplessness has far-reaching effects. In 1977, Madelon Visintainer, one of Seligman's graduate students, performed an experiment showing how mastery and helplessness affect health. She put three groups of rats through the same shock experiment as Seligman had with the dogs, but with an important addition. The day before the experiment she implanted a few cancer cells on each rat's flank. Under normal conditions, 50% of the rats would reject the cancer cells and live. As expected, 50% of the rats who were not shocked had died, and the other half had rejected the tumor. Of the rats who were allowed to escape the shock by pressing a bar, the rats who had learned mastery, 70% rejected the tumor. But only 27% of the helpless rats, the rats who had experienced uncontrollable shock, rejected the cancer cells. In short, Visintainer became the first person to demonstrate that the psychological state of helplessness produces a more rapid growth of cancer. She also showed, of course, that the psychological state of mastery enhances the ability to reject the tumor. And that's not all. Visintainer went on to demonstrate that the rats who had experienced mastery when young were better protected against tumors as adults.

Learned Optimism

Seligman says it works the same way in humans. Researchers at Yale found that elderly people in nursing homes were not only happier when they were given greater control over the daily happenings in their lives, but they also lived longer. As noted earlier, optimists have better immune activity than pessimists. For example, Seligman and his colleagues taught learned optimism to 40 cancer patients and produced a very sharp increase in the activity of natural killer cells, the cells that kill foreign invaders in the body, such as viruses, bacteria and tumor cells.

So, the emphasis you and your son place on attitude is well founded.

Your view of bodybuilding, I believe, is correct as well. I started lifting weights at 12 or 13, and I believe it gave me a positive outlook on life, an optimistic frame of reference that has persisted.

Weight training taught me that what I did counted, that I had the power to shape the course of my life. I was small for my age and I think I felt a little inferior. I wanted to change that, and I did. I wanted to be as strong as — no, stronger than — my school buddies. Through weight training, I not only eclipsed my friends, I surpassed them. As a junior I won the state high school pentathlon championship, a five-event contest consisting of push-ups, chin-ups, jump reach, bar vault and 300-yard shuttle run. A short time later I became city, state and regional champion in the Olympic lifts. In short, weight training taught me that if I set realistic goals and worked hard, I would succeed. Those early successes taught me that perseverance pays. They set the pattern for the rest of my life, a pattern which has extended far beyond sports. For instance, the stick-to-ittiveness that I learned through weight training helped me graduate second in my class from a law school that flunked four out of five entering students. And it has helped me in everything I've attempted since then.

Yes, you're right! Bodybuilding is a can-do sport. It does much more than build muscle and fitness. It makes you an optimistic person, one who can bounce back from life's inevitable setbacks again and again.

FEAR NO MORE!

To maintain your enthusiasm, you've got to leave some room for enjoyment

I was between a rock and a hard place. The 1992 Mile High Indoor Rowing Classic was less than a month away, and I had a decision to make. It boiled down to this: how much physical and emotional pain was I willing to endure?

Let me give you some background. In 1990 and '91, I had entered the annual indoor regatta on Concept II Rowing Ergometers staged by the Rocky Mountain Rowing Club in Denver. The event is a regional qualifying trial for the World Indoor Rowing Championships. However, most competitors, like me, are "mere mortals" who simply want the satisfaction that comes from doing our best.

That was part of my problem. In 1990, I achieved a personal record for 2500 meters and placed seventh in the Veteran Men's category. Last year I improved my time by nine seconds and moved up to second in my age group. So I knew that it would take a major effort to top myself again this year. Plus, my preparation was behind schedule because of an elbow injury. But the recovery and the hard training I faced weren't my only problems. It was far more complicated than that.

My column in the August 1990 *Muscle & Fitness* described the physical and psychological obstacles I've encountered in training for rowing competition. During hard rowing sessions, as I fought to get my breath, I sometimes felt like I was suffocating, sort of a feeling of impending doom. During computerized interval workouts I often felt like I was trapped on a merciless mechanical monster. In short, I developed a major aversion to the pain and discomfort that are inevitable parts of an all-out row, especially the 2500-meter competitive distance.

Apparently, my experience is not unique, because a short time after my column appeared, I received a wonderful letter from a worldclass "on-the-water" oarsman. Tommie Weling, a member of the 1988 U.S. Olympic rowing team who also rowed for the University of Washington Huskies when they won two national championships, identified so completely with the feelings I described that he felt compelled to write. Weling, now in his 30s and a real estate broker, said he currently does his rowing indoors on the Concept II. Interestingly, his new passion is bodybuilding.

Self-Induced Torture?

"Your feelings of impending doom are very real," Weling wrote. "Rowing is so much self-induced torture that you often ask yourself why you do it." Unfortunately, he continued, "the feelings never change, nor do they leave you.

"Do not feel that you are alone or that your fear of 'hitting the wall' or stopping during hard rowing is anything but very ordinary. Every (rower) feels the same fear, breathlessness and panic."

He added, however, that "it's those who can control and conquer that anxiety and push forward, letting the body experience what can be the most agonizing 10 minutes you could imagine, who get the rush and feeling of confidence and mastery at the end of a race or ergometer piece."

He concluded with these encouraging words: "Stick with it. Rowing is a sport you can excel at forever. You have already begun to master your most formidable enemy: your own mind."

So that's the background. Here's the rest of the story:

As the competition approached and my rowing workouts became more intense, the feelings of impending doom returned. About three minutes into a 2500-meter trial, I stopped rowing. The problem was not physical. I was maintaining the pace with no particular difficulty. It was mental. I just could not handle the thought of another seven minutes of hard rowing, especially the agony of the final 500 meters.

I was at a crossroads. What to do? Should I pass on the rowing

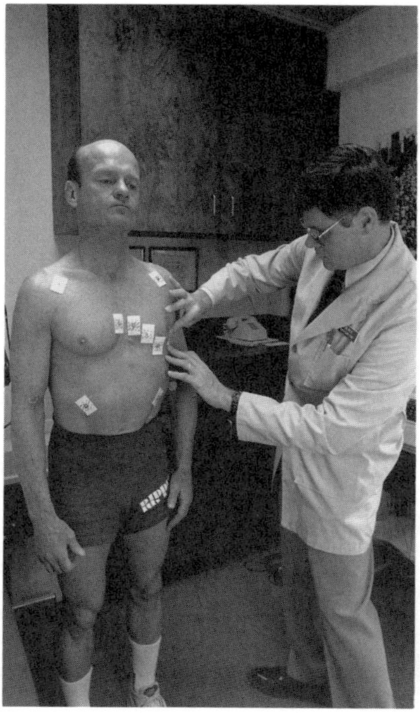

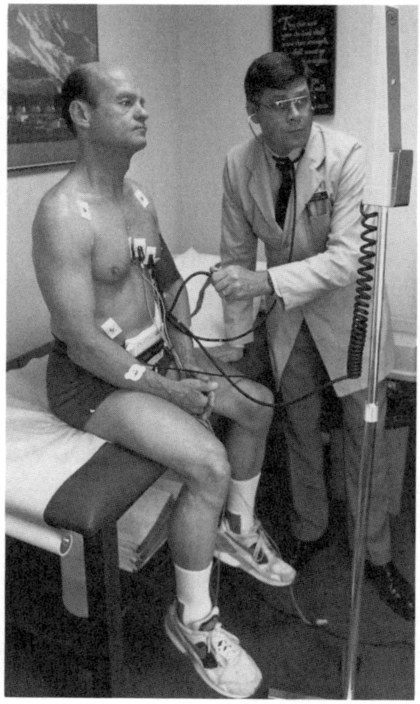

Getting wired up at the Cooper Clinic for my latest treadmill test. *Photos by Justin Joseph.*

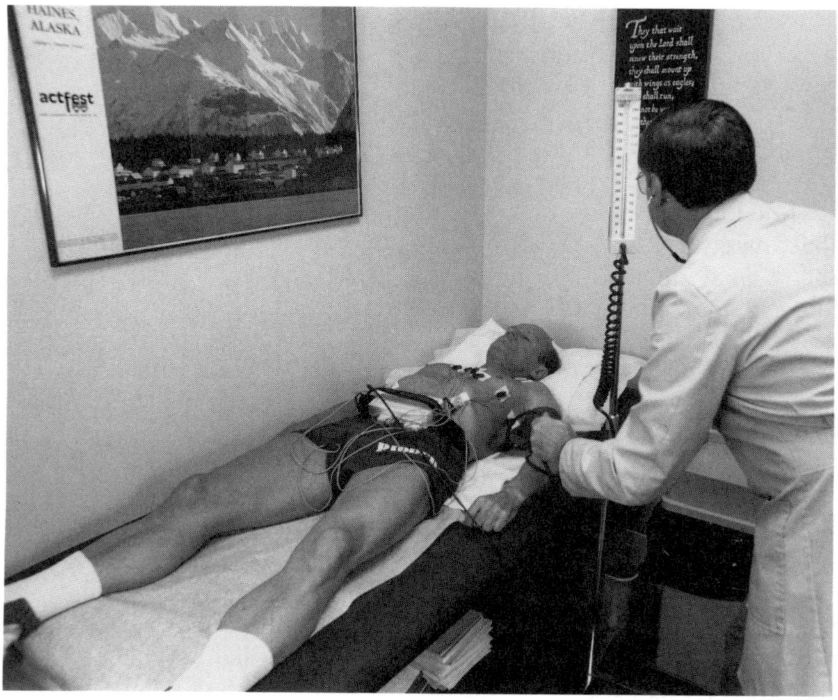

competition? Should I try to overcome my fears and push on for a new personal record? Or was there some middle ground?

I had lunch and then went for a long walk. Walking often helps me come up with a logical solution. I decided to continue rowing because, frankly, I really like the rowing motion. It feels good — that is, if it's not carried too far. I enjoy a hard rowing session, but I don't like being forced to suffer beyond a certain point. I don't like being in a situation where I feel like I have to continue whether I want to or not.

I decided to enter the competition, but with an important attitude adjustment. I decided that I would train hard, but I would also give myself permission to back off or even stop rowing, if necessary. That made a big difference in how I approached each workout. I no longer awoke on the day of a rowing workout with that suffocating feeling. I decided that I was going to enjoy my workouts. Finally, I decided that I would row as hard as I could in Denver, but that I would not feel compelled to make a new PR.

Satisfied

To make a long story short, I did compete in Denver. And even though my time was 15 seconds slower than last year's, I was satisfied with my effort. I didn't give up, and I was rowing as hard as I could at the end of the race. My time was 9:52.6, which put me third out of 11 over-50 rowers in terms of raw score. When the age handicap was plugged in, I dropped to eighth.

Importantly, I didn't burn myself out. I returned home still enthusiastic about rowing. In fact, I decided to continue rowing for a few more weeks and try to post a better time before the March 1 deadline for the 1992 Concept II World Ranking. As I write this I am enjoying my rowing workouts — and improving. I feel confident that I can improve on my time in Denver. After all, that's what training is really all about, improving on your recent best and having fun in the process.

I do not mean to imply, of course, that I have overcome my fear of a maximum effort on the Concept II rower. As Tommie Weling said, that never goes away. I simply called a shaky truce with myself. I cut myself some slack, so to speak — just enough to ensure that I will keep rowing and continue to enjoy it. As Dr. George Sheehan has written, "exercise should not be like the medicine we down as we hold our nose to minimize the taste and smell... It should be a reward — a time set apart to enjoy alone or with others."

Exercise and athletic competition — rowing, bodybuilding, whatever — can easily become just one more stress in an already stress-filled life. It was a close call, but I finally decided not to let that happen with my rowing. Why not follow my lead? When you go to the gym, be sure to set the dial on "fun."

FEAR OF FRYING

A simple — and effective — coping strategy for peak performance

I believe it was Vince Lombardi who said, "Fatigue makes cowards of us all." In my case, that was true before my second treadmill test at the Cooper Aerobics Center in Dallas in 1989. Actually, it was my memory of the first test that made me fearful.

When I was tested the first time, in 1988, I didn't know what to expect. I simply got on the treadmill and did my best, without a lot of worry beforehand. Dr. Arnie Jensen, the doctor who invited me to come to the center for testing, said I would do well, and I believed him. As it turned out, he was right. My time, 28 minutes, put me above the 99th percentile for men 50-59 and in the "superior" category for men under 30.

But 1989 was different. I knew what was coming only too well. I knew the test was absolutely unforgiving. As you grow more fatigued, the test gets harder. The angle of incline goes up 1% each minute to 25%, and after that the speed increases every minute. As David Prokop wrote after my first test (*M&F*, May 1989), "A treadmill test to exhaustion is a journey to nowhere in which the destination isn't a place, but a physical state: total fatigue — or as close to total fatigue as you can get."

So you can understand why I was apprehensive before the second test. I vividly remember tossing and turning in bed before the test, thinking — over and over — about the final minutes of the test, those unrelenting speedups on the way to total exhaustion. I was up and down all night, and when I finally stepped on the treadmill my blood pressure, as recorded by the exercise technician, was sky-high. In short, the period leading up to the second test was a nightmare.

Even though I again did well (29 minutes), I told Jensen I would not be back the next year. I needed a break — to get my head on straight, so to speak — before subjecting myself to another test.

As it turned out, I waited three years, until November 1992, when I turned 55. This was sufficient time to rethink my mental approach to the dreaded treadmill test. Plus, three years is long enough to assess whether I am declining with age. Conventional wisdom, of course, says I should lose about 3% of my physical capacity in that time.

Biggest Hurdle

The fear of working to exhaustion

My biggest hurdle was coping with the fear of driving myself to exhaustion. Flipping TV channels recently, I caught the end of an interview with a psychotherapist on the subject of fear. I didn't get his name, but I wrote down a very perceptive comment. "Fear," he said, "is a dark room where negatives develop." That's true, isn't it? As Terry Orlick, Ph.D., has written, "Worry raises anxiety, drains energy, and diminishes your performance focus" (*In Pursuit of Excellence,* Leisure Press, second edition, 1990). Intellectually, at least, we all realize that fear and worry are counterproductive. I certainly know that. Still, the problem remained: how could I avoid, or at least mitigate, my very real and human fear of the treadmill test?

I decided on a long- and short-term approach to the problem. From the long-term standpoint, I prepared myself physically. This is just common sense. We all have less fear and anxiety when we know we are well prepared for the task at hand. I mapped out a training plan early on and stuck with it. As the saying goes, "I planned my work and worked my plan." Without going into detail, I felt good about my training. I knew I was capable of posting a good time.

That kept me in a positive frame of mind until a few weeks before the test, when my fear level started to rise again. As the test grew near it became obvious that I had to work on my attitude — or repeat the miserable 1989 experience. I needed a way to deal with my fear. With the help of *In Pursuit of Excellence,* I decided on a simple — and effective — coping strategy.

Fear does not exist outside your head. Situations are not anxious, *people* are. I could not change the fact that the treadmill test would be brutally hard, but I could control the way I thought about it. As I've said, I was prepared. I knew I would do well when I finally got on the treadmill. I had a job to do, and I knew I was capable of doing it. I decided to do my best. Beyond that, I resolved to stop worrying about it. Moreover, I reminded myself that the worry is almost always worse than the event itself. Shakespeare, in *Julius Caesar,* said, "Cowards die many times before their deaths; The valiant never taste of death but once."

Short-Term Strategy

Relax, focus, be confident

My short-term strategy boiled down to three simple reminders: Relax. Focus. Be confident. I thought of these cue words every time I started to feel anxious about the test. In other words, I developed a specific response to my fear.

"Relax" reminded me to take a deep breath and be calm. "Focus" reminded me to stay in the moment. It's hard to be anxious about something in the future, if you are fully absorbed in what you're doing at the time. "Be confident" told me to encourage myself, tell myself that I am well prepared and capable of doing a good job. I had my wife Carol type the cue words on a card, which I carried in my pocket. I didn't actually take the card out very often, but it was reassuring to

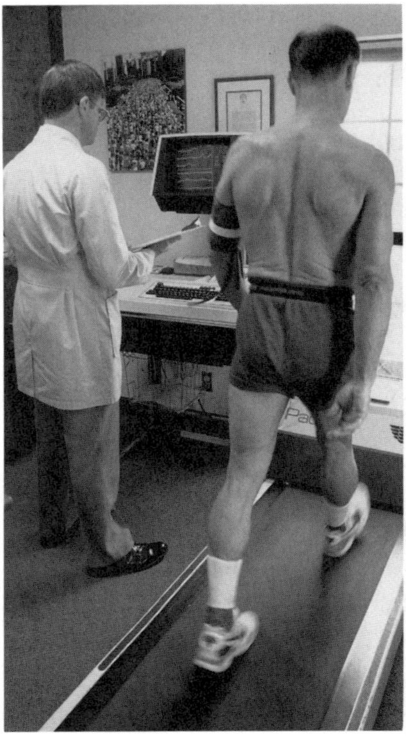

"Here we go."

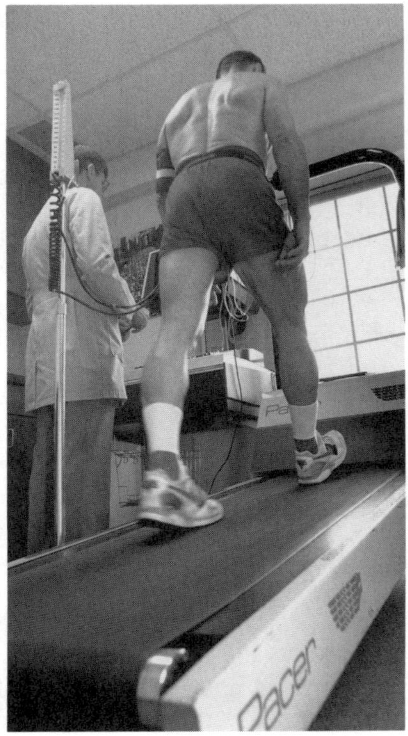

"Getting harder now."

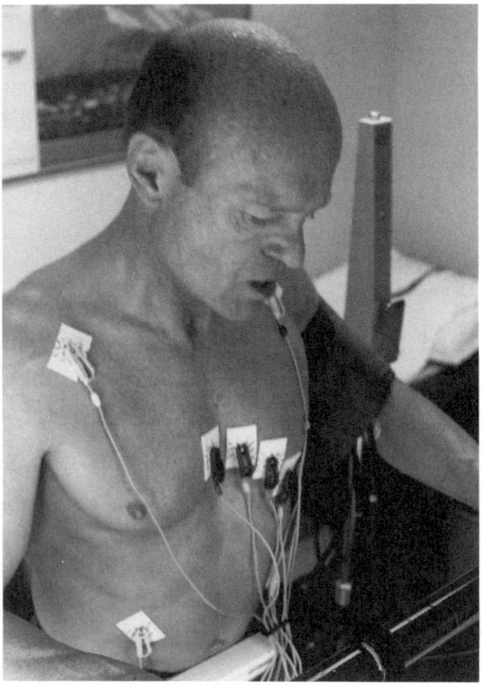

"Thank God, it's over. My strategy worked!" *Photo by Justin Joseph.*

know it was there. The minute I started to feel anxious, I used the cue words to trigger my prepared response. This worked surprisingly well.

I managed to avoid worrying about the test until almost the moment I stepped on the treadmill. I read a book on the flight to Dallas. In the room that night, I occupied myself watching television and reading magazines I had carefully selected before leaving home. The magazines contained articles of interest to me, but ones that would not trigger my anxiety; for example, none were sports related. I can't say I slept very well that night, but I didn't think about the treadmill test.

The next morning I continued to focus on what I was doing at the time. This was easy to do, because Jensen kept me busy with this test and that one until the time for the treadmill finally arrived.

I used basically the same strategy for the test itself. I focused on the present, because that's all I could control. I did not let my mind think ahead. I took each minute as it came. I focused on doing my job, and when the crunch came — those final few minutes before exhaustion —I did my best.

My time was 28.38. This placed me at the 99.5th percentile among the 6,816 males, age 50-59, who had been tested at the center through October 1992. My performance, again, placed me in the top category for men under 30.

Finally, I was especially pleased that I achieved a maximum heart rate of 190 beats per minute. This is significant because the rule of thumb is that maximum heart rate declines one beat per year, even for those who continue to train hard. The expected decline must not be inevitable, because in my two previous tests my maximum heart rate was recorded at 183, seven beats less than this time around. That tells me two things. My coping strategy worked; fear did not prevent me from doing my best. Happily, it also suggests that Father Time is treating me well.

CHAPTER NINE

HEALTH FACTORS

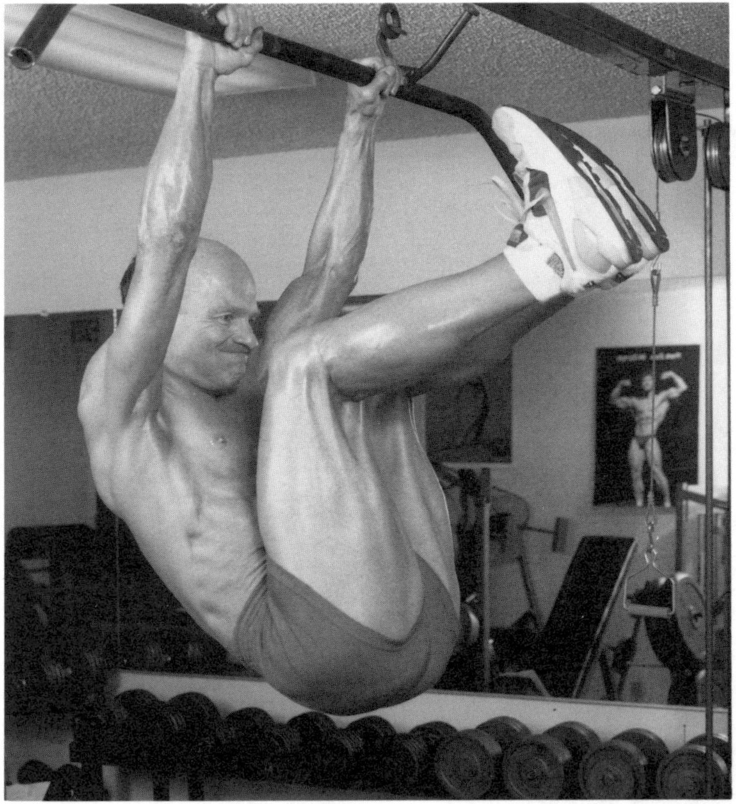

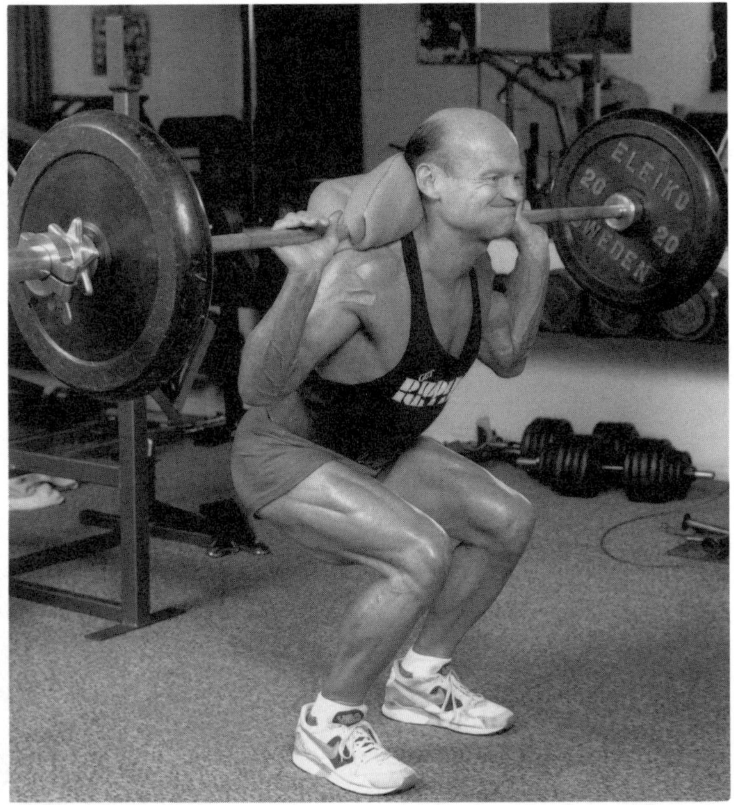

Photos by Pat Berrett.

HEALTH FACTORS 9

THE LIFESTYLE DISEASE

You can prevent diverticulosis

It may be unclear whether heart rate decline can be slowed, but there's one age-related malady that most of us can prevent. That's diverticulosis — the ruptures, or blow-outs, of the wall of the colon that occur in one-half to two-thirds of our senior citizens.

Until the early 1900s, diverticulosis was virtually unknown. Your ancestors probably didn't have it, but I'll bet you know someone today who does. So what brought about the change?

It's pretty simple, really. We stopped eating whole foods, foods with roughage, and switched to refined products such as white flour, which have the fiber removed. That's why diverticulosis is sometimes called "the miller's revenge."

Here's how it works: the large intestine, the colon, works best when it contains plenty of bulk. The movement of food residue along the colon is accomplished by a series of rhythmic contractions. The colon needs bulk to do its job properly. When the colon is not adequately filled, it has to contract more and harder. This results in hard, dry stools, and over many years the increased force of contractions creates enough pressure to cause little ruptures or balloons in the wall of the colon.

Some people have diverticulosis and never know it. Others, however, have severe symptoms. Fecal matter passes into the little ruptures and causes inflammation. When this happens, it's called diverticulitis. The result is pain and fever, and in severe cases bleeding and even perforation of the intestine.

As I've suggested, this is a lifestyle disease. It can usually be prevented by eating plenty of whole grains, fresh fruits and vegetables. In other words, the foods that I recommended in my books and in this column to become and stay lean also prevent diverticulosis.

This added benefit of the *Ripped* diet was graphically confirmed in the course of the complete medical and fitness evaluation I underwent last year at the Cooper Clinic.

The Cooper Clinic examined the entire length of my colon fluoroscopically and by X-ray. I was actually able to see all five feet or so of my colon as the examination was taking place. The results were completely negative. I have no sign of diverticulosis.

So take it from me — I saw it with my own eyes — eating right pays big dividends.

CATCH-22

Break the connection between arthritis & obesity

Q: *My father and I are both overweight. My father is about 70 pounds heavier than he should be, and I'm 80-90 pounds overweight. We realize the importance of exercise in losing weight, but we both have arthritis, which limits our physical activity. My father has a bad back and even worse knees. He's been on a walking program, but when I try to encourage him to exercise more, he replies that it's difficult because of his bad knees.*

I've been walking and also doing more strenuous activities. The additional activity has helped me lose some weight, but, like my father, I'm unable to be as active as I'd like. Are there any exercises that will help us lose weight, but not put a great deal of stress on the joints?

A: To lose weight, of course, you've got to watch your diet, taking in fewer calories than you burn. But it's true that exercise is a vital part of any reducing program. You and your father are quite perceptive. Your arthritis keeps you from being active enough to lose weight, and your excess weight aggravates your arthritis. It's a Catch-22 situation. Still, there's hope for you yet. And your case should be of interest to other readers because almost everyone has some evidence of osteoarthritis (a degeneration of the cartilage, which can cause pain and disability in the joints) by age 40 or 50.

Obesity & Arthritis

First, you are correct that obesity and arthritis go hand in hand. This was demonstrated in the Framingham study on obesity and knee osteoarthritis (*Ann Intern Med* 1988; 109: 18-24). This study, which continued for more than 35 years, found a strong relationship between obesity at an early age and the development of arthritis in the knees when you get older. The researchers concluded that obesity is probably an important cause of osteoarthritis of the knee.

This makes sense because as Lawrence E. Lamb, MD, observed recently in *The Health Letter*: "When you are walking, the knee is subjected to three times the body weight. That means even small losses of body weight will be of great benefit to the arthritic knee."

The actual cause of osteoarthritis is not completely understood, according to Lamb. Nevertheless, he says, "We know that injury or improper overuse of joints may contribute to its early development."

So, as your letter indicates, exercise can aggravate an arthritic condition, especially if you're overweight.

This presents a dilemma, because, as a practical matter, it's almost impossible to control your bodyfat level without regular exercise. As I wrote in *Ripped 3*: "The more active you are, the leaner you're likely to be. That seems to be nature's way. Your body tends to mirror your lifestyle."

All Is Not Lost

Nevertheless, as I've already suggested, all is not lost for you and your father. A carefully crafted program of weight training and aerobic exercise should allow you to lose weight without aggravating your arthritis. Moreover, it will probably relieve your arthritic symptoms as well.

You and your father will have to see a physical therapist or sports-medicine physician for help in developing individualized exercise routines. I can give you some guidelines here, however.

First, weight training can prevent pain by developing muscles that support your joints. Strong muscles act as shock absorbers, deflecting energy from the joint. As I said in *The Lean Advantage 2,* paraphrasing Dr. Robert P. Nirschl, assistant professor of orthopedic surgery at Georgetown University School of Medicine: "It's like jumping off a platform with your knees flexed as opposed to having them locked. With your knees bent the leg muscles — not your joints — absorb the shock."

The trick, of course, is to strengthen the muscles without aggravating your arthritis. The main thing is to stick to lighter weights and higher reps (15 or more) and do smooth, steady motions. Don't jerk! Tense your muscles hard at the end of each repetition. This way you can overload and strengthen your muscles without unduly stressing the joints. Don't copy powerlifters and Olympic lifters, who try to lift as much weight as possible; they have many more joint problems than bodybuilders, who use less weight and higher reps.

I suggest that you and your father try training with weights about twice a week. Stick with a few basic exercises and train your whole body each session.

That will give you five days rest from the weights. That's important, because according to *The Health Letter* Special Report 80, there is one fundamental truth: "All joints afflicted with osteoarthritis improve if they are rested."

Rest Is Important

This basic rule, that rest is important for arthritis sufferers, should also be your guiding light in aerobic exercise. You must derive the fat-burning benefits of aerobic exercise without overstressing your tender joints.

As with weight training, avoid jerking and jarring your joints. In addition, wear shoes that cushion your feet when you walk and avoid running on hard surfaces.

Stick with smooth, nonjarring activities like biking and rowing. The adjustable treadmills found in most gyms are also good. They offer smooth, steady exercise that minimizes the stress on arthritic joints. By raising the angle of the treadmill, you can get a terrific workout just walking; there's no need to pound your joints by running.

My next suggestion is very important. Your program should include aerobic exercise for the upper body. That's because spreading aerobic exercise over your upper as well as your lower body will help you avoid overstressing individual joints. I'll give you an example of how this works.

In his later years, my father had a weak and atrophied leg. He also had arthritis in both shoulders. In spite of these problems, he was able to use the Schwinn Air-Dyne, a stationary bicycle which includes a push-pull arm action. With the Air-Dyne, his three good limbs made up for the weakness of his bad leg, and his arthritis shoulders tolerated the smooth arm action well.

Many Exercise Machines

I suggest that you and your father investigate the Air-Dyne and the other whole-body aerobic exercise machines now on the market. Rowing machines have been available for a long time. Cross-country ski machines such as the NordicTrack work both the upper and lower body, and provide smooth, even resistance. And then there's the VersaClimber, which provides a smooth climbing action using both the arms and legs. In some gyms you'll even find stationary bicycles that you pump with your arms. The Air-Dyne, VersaClimber and NordicTrack can also be used with the arms alone.

With all the aerobic exercise machines now available, it's possible to exercise your whole body in many different ways. You and your father should take advantage of this variety. You'll probably find a number of motions you can tolerate quite well. Plus, the variety will allow you to exercise one part of your body while resting another. As I've said, that's extremely important for arthritis sufferers; your only sure relief is rest.

I'm optimistic that these suggestions will allow you and your father to exercise more and lose bodyfat. And relieved of 70-90 excess pounds, your arthritic joints will be in seventh heaven. Plus, as I mentioned earlier, there's evidence that exercise itself may relieve your arthritic symptoms.

The February 1989 issue of *The Physician and Sportsmedicine* contained a review of the research on arthritis and aerobic exercise. It concluded that aerobic exercise for arthritis sufferers can have "a positive impact on pain tolerance, joint pain, mood, and social activity." I urge you to read the details for yourself.

The bottom line is that an intelligent, varied exercise program *including adequate rest* will do the job for you and your father. You'll be stronger, leaner and fitter. You'll look better, and you'll feel better — all over.

I should close with some cautionary notes, however:

1) Include warm-up and cool-down exercises in both your weight training and aerobic exercise programs.

2) Contact your physician before you plunge into a new exercise program; he or she knows the specific details of your disability and can alert you to possible pitfalls.

3) Finally, I'll repeat the advice I gave arthritis sufferers in *The Lean Advantage 2*: "If it hurts, don't do it."

THE FITNESS PAY-OFF

People who exercise live longer

Q: *Your wife Carol said you would be happy to help an overweight dentist get started on the road to improved fitness. Here's my situation.*

I'll be 40 in June. My weight is at an all-time high, 230. I estimate my bodyfat to be about 28%. I'm 6'1" and my waist is 42. My diet has been a typical fat person's diet: beer, pizza, ice cream, Mexican food, hamburgers, fries and the like.

Over the years, my weight's been creeping upward, despite occasional weight-loss attempts, and my exercise involvement has declined, especially since I twisted my knee five months ago. I've been to the Cooper Clinic four times and my treadmill times have been declining.

Why am I contacting you now? Last week when I held my 5-day-old adopted son for the first time, I knew I had to make some major changes in my life or I wouldn't be around to see him grow into an adult! At the airport that evening, I picked up a copy of Muscle & Fitness *and read your column. I realized that your method — weight training, diet and aerobics — was what I needed. I ordered your books the very next day. Do you have any additional advice?*

A: I hear from many people who at about your age decide they'd better start taking care of their bodies. A lawyer friend of mine who specializes in estate planning says there comes a point when people

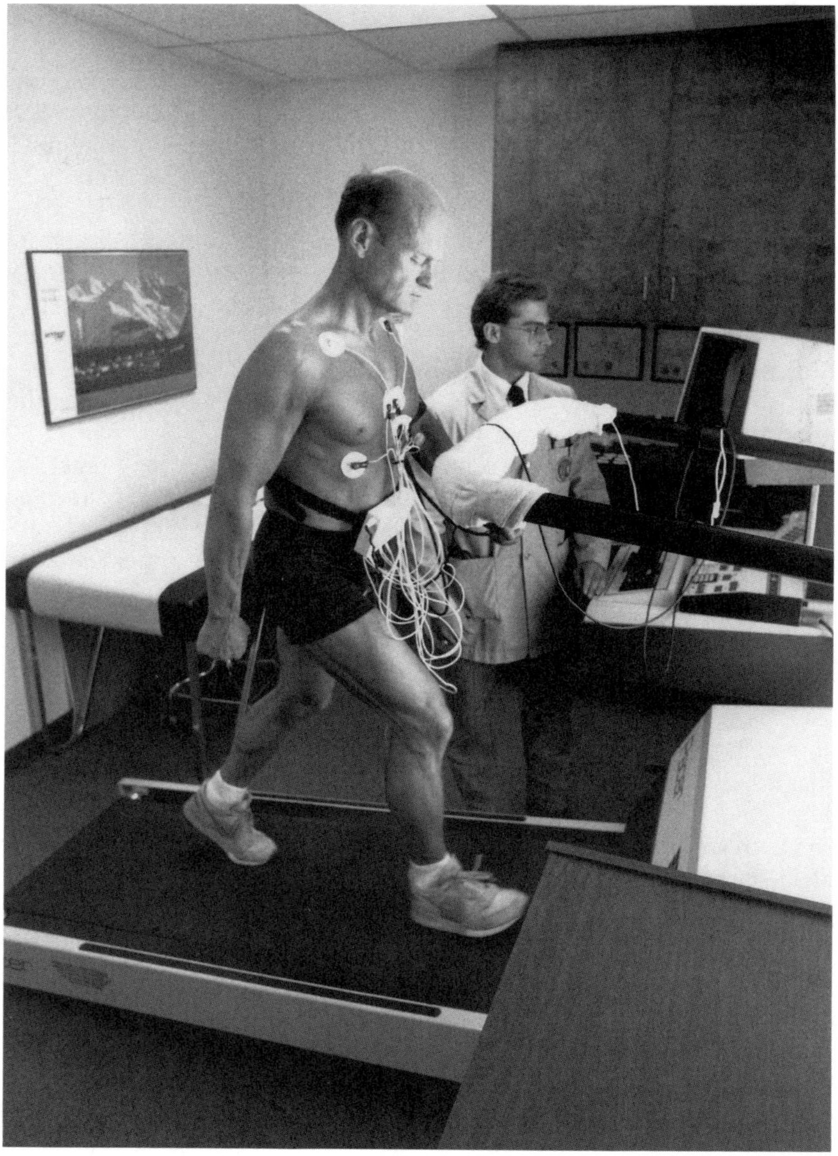

This was taken during my first treadmill test at the Cooper Clinic in 1988. *Photo by Justin Joseph.*

stop talking about "if" they die and switch to "when." In our 20s we think we'll live forever. At about 40 it dawns on us that maybe we're not indestructible after all. People come to this realization by different routes. In your case a new baby at 39 spurred you to action.

A just-published study on the relationship between physical fitness and mortality will make you even more enthusiastic about getting in shape.

Fitness Study

This study shows that regular exercise will significantly increase your chances of being around to see your son grow into manhood. What's more, you don't have to spend hours in the gym or become a topnotch triathlete. Even a minimal amount of exercise — a brisk 30-45 minute walk each day is enough — protects you against premature death.

In the past, you plunged into diets and exercise programs you were not able to maintain. You bit off more than you could chew. This study shows that a more moderate, more realistic program — one you can stick to — is just what the doctor ordered for a business professional and family man like you. The study was published in the Nov. 3, 1989 *Journal of the American Medical Association.* Here are the details.

The Institute for Aerobic Research in Dallas (better known as the Cooper Clinic) followed 10,224 men and 3,120 women who were given a preventive medical examination, including a maximal treadmill test, between 1970 and 1981. After their exam, these 13,344 men and women were followed for an average of more than eight years. At the end of that time, 240 men and 43 women, all of whom were in good health when initially examined, had died. The subjects were placed in five fitness categories based on their treadmill performance. The 20% with the lowest treadmill times were classified as unfit; the top 20% were classified as highly fit; and those in the middle were classified as moderately fit.

The researchers found that men in the first group, the least fit, were 3.44 times as likely to die early as the most fit men. The least fit women were 4.65 times more likely to die than those in the best shape.

Common sense says that fit people should live longer than couch potatoes. This study proves it. Even after weeding out other risk factors, including smoking, age, cholesterol levels, weight, blood pressure and family history of heart disease, the researchers found that deaths were sharply higher in the least-fit category than in the moderately fit group — more than double for men and almost twice as high for women.

A Little Exercise Helps A Lot

Importantly, those in the high-fitness group were only slightly less likely to die than those in the medium-fitness groups. In short, you don't have to be superfit to greatly reduce your mortality. Even moderate fitness affords significant protection not only from cardiovascular disease and cancer but also against death from a wide range of other causes. *Simply put, people who exercise even moderately tend to live longer.*

It's Up To You

So there's the evidence. Now it's up to you. I suggest that you start out moderately. Don't go overboard, as I suspect you have in the past. Read about the diet and exercise programs detailed in my books. Then make changes in your lifestyle that you know you can live with comfortably. Again, don't bite off more than you can chew. If you're comfortable with your diet and exercise program, you'll be happy to stay with it for the rest of your life.

My friend Dr. Arnie Jensen, a preventive medicine specialist at the Cooper Clinic, says that people would like to have a pill which will improve their health and fitness and make them look and feel better. "That pill is available now," he says. "It just takes longer — about 30 minutes — to swallow it four times a week." The pill to which he refers, of course, is exercise. Elaborating, Jensen says, "Health is 50% lifestyle, 10% medicine, and the rest genetics and luck."

Those are words to live by. Jensen knows his stuff. The landmark study by Dr. Kenneth Cooper and his colleagues proves it. Fitness has a big payoff: longer life.

WEIGHTS & LIFESTYLE

Done correctly, weight training lowers blood pressure

Q: *I'm 47 and for the last couple of years have been experimenting with various weightlifting routines. Over the last couple of months I've made especially good progress. I do primarily power movements. I also try to do aerobics four days a week, but this has been sporadic of late.*

My bodyweight has increased about 10% — mostly muscle, I hope, but some of it's probably fat.

The fly in the ointment is my blood pressure. When I began lifting about two years ago, it was 110/70. It has recently gone up, however; my latest reading was 140/90. I'd like to get my blood pressure back down and improve my bench by about 30%.

What suggestions do you have?

A: I have a number of suggestions, including a revamp of your exercise program. You must discuss them with your doctor, however. This is important because your blood pressure is at a level where physicians start to become concerned. The generally accepted borderline hypertension level begins at 140/90.

New Rule Of Thumb

The old rule of thumb was that your systolic (upper) blood pressure should be no higher than 100 plus your age. Using this approach, a pressure reading up to 147 would have been acceptable for you. In his book *Overcoming Hypertension* (Bantam Books, 1990), Kenneth H. Cooper, MD, disagrees with the 100-plus-your-age approach. "I've discovered that exercise and a healthy diet and lifestyle can keep the average person's blood pressure near the levels of youth," says Cooper. He and his colleagues at the Aerobics Institute in Dallas have shown this with surveys involving generally fit men of different ages who maintain a healthy lifestyle. For example, in a survey of nearly 100 men under age 30 the median blood pressure was 120/78. Another survey of more than 3,200 men age 50-59 revealed that the median blood pressure was only 125/82. Furthermore, a survey of more than 1,000 men over age 60 showed their median blood pressure was 132/82. As you can see, the readings increased very little even though the age of those surveyed more than doubled.

So your doctor will probably want to investigate the cause or causes of your slightly elevated blood pressure, and help you restore your excellent pressure readings of a few years ago.

Transitory Elevation

Your physician may also be concerned about your heavy weightlifting. According to Cooper, weight training is potentially dangerous if you have high blood pressure. Strenuous weightlifting can cause a major rise in blood pressure, at least temporarily. Dr. Duncan MacDougall of the department of physical education and medicine at McMaster University in Hamilton, Ontario, Canada, measured the average blood pressure of experienced bodybuilders (*The Physician and Sportsmedicine,* July 1984). A series of leg presses produced an average blood pressure level of 355/281. One-arm curls caused an average pressure of 293/230. These were, of course, transitory elevations. Most people can tolerate temporary increases in blood pressure, but MacDougall expressed concern that heavy weightlifting by hypertensive individuals may be dangerous.

This doesn't mean, of course, that weight training causes hypertension. In fact, my own example suggests just the opposite. I've been lifting heavy weights for almost 40 years, and my blood pressure is the same as when I was a teenager. Dr. Arnie Jensen, at the time of my physical examination last year at the Cooper Clinic, called my pressure readings "absolutely superb."

How Weights Help

Jensen, a preventive medicine specialist, says weight training, done properly, helps your blood pressure because it develops the small blood vessels, especially in the often neglected upper body area. In fact, no other form of exercise systematically trains all the muscles — and the

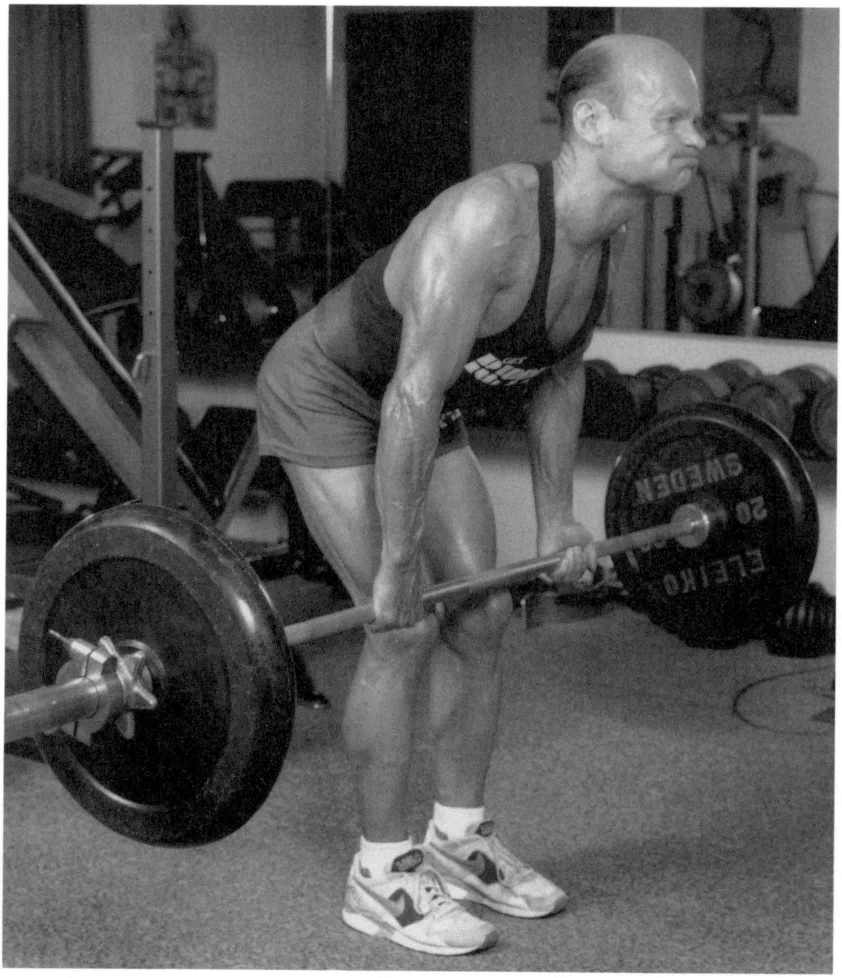

The Cooper Clinic says my blood pressure is "absolutely superb." *Photo by Pat Berrett.*

blood vessels — in the body like bodybuilding. In untrained individuals, the small veins and arteries are constricted or closed, which leads to high blood pressure. Weight training opens these small blood pathways, Jensen explains. The effect is like increasing the diameter of your garden hose: the pressure drops.

An important caveat is that these benefits are attained in those who do more than just a few near-maximum contractions and quit. As I explained in *Ripped 3,* best results come from doing 8-20 repetitions. That's the range most bodybuilders use. And listen up: Very low reps are not the best way to build strength either. If you perform less than six or eight repetitions you probably won't exhaust a high percentage of muscle fibers. Low repetitions may be good for *testing* strength, but they're not the best way to build muscle size *or* strength.

Fred Hatfield, the former world champion powerlifter who has squatted with more than 1,000 pounds, agrees: "Even powerlifters are learning that maximum singles in training do not help them get stronger over the long term. Most powerlifters have retreated, so to speak, to the 5-8-reps-per-set method for strength training, leaving the singles for the contest."

Don't Hold Your Breath

I suggest that you drop your low-repetition sets. You'll make better progress on your bench press, and you'll also be less likely to push your blood pressure to dangerous levels. Very high pressure readings come when you hold your breath and strain for long periods of time. As you know, that's most likely to happen when you lift very heavy weights for one or two reps. With lighter weights and eight or more repetitions, it's easier to control your breathing. For people with elevated blood pressure, and even for those with normal pressure, it's important to breathe when you lift. I know it's necessary to hold your breath momentarily during a hard rep, but if you concentrate you can breathe regularly throughout most of a set. It also helps to relax briefly between repetitions. This gives the blood a chance to circulate. And here's a point Jensen emphasizes: don't grab the bar with a death grip. Again, breathe and relax while you lift.

Finally, according to the *Harvard Medical School Health Letter,* hypertension is a disease of civilized life. Most people can lower their blood pressure by adjusting their lifestyle. That usually means eliminating excess bodyfat, not smoking, eliminating or limiting alcohol intake, limiting sodium intake, following a good exercise program and reducing stress. I believe you're already doing most of the right things, but I'd like to comment on two points.

Primary Risk Factor

First, you say you may have gained some fat. That may account for part of your rise in blood pressure. Being overweight may be the *primary* factor contributing to hypertension, according to Cooper. Nobody knows exactly why this is so, but Cooper says one possibility is that an increase in weight brings with it an increase in blood volume and in the force with which the heart pumps blood. In short, weight gain makes your heart work harder, which increases your blood pressure. So clearly one thing you should do is lose the fat.

You admit to not being regular in your aerobic exercise. I feel sure your doctor would scold you about that. Hear Cooper: "Regular aerobic exercise — such as jogging, running, cycling, and swimming — is one of the most effective non-drug 'medicines' for those at risk for hypertension." Without question you should be consistent in your aerobic exercise. As a bonus, regular aerobics will help you lose the fat you've gained.

OPEN THOSE ARTERIES!

The best way to get ripped — and prevent heart disease

Q: *I'm sure many of us would be interested in how your current training and low-fat/high-fiber diet has affected your total cholesterol and high-density-lipoprotein cholesterol levels.*

A: My inclination has always been to do whatever it takes to get lean and muscular. It just so happens that experience and study have taught me that the best way to get ripped *and stay ripped* is also the best way to prevent heart disease. That's becoming clearer every day. A study just published in the British medical journal *The Lancet* helps make my point. This study shows that mild exercise and a stringent diet, without drugs, can not only halt heart disease but reverse it.

The Lifestyle Heart Trial directed by Dean Ornish, MD, head of the Preventive Medicine Research Institute, Sausalito, California and on the faculty of the University of California, San Francisco School of Medicine, is an ongoing study to determine whether lifestyle changes alone — no drugs, no surgery — can not only slow or stop the progress of heart disease but actually open clogged arteries. The study produced the first hard evidence that the answer is yes. Here are the exciting details.

Exciting Study Results

A total of 48 patients with documented coronary artery disease (computer enhanced X-rays showed that their heart arteries were partially blocked) were divided into experimental and control groups. Significantly, all of these people were already restricting fat intake to 30% of total calories, as usually recommended for heart disease patients. The patients (28) in the experimental group were put on an extremely low fat diet (10%) and given minimal exercise and stress management. The remaining 20 patients, the control group, were not asked to make lifestyle changes.

The diet eaten by the experimental group included fruits, vegetables, grains, legumes and soybean products without calorie restrictions. No animal products were allowed except egg whites and one cup per day of nonfat milk or yogurt. The diet contained about 10% fat calories, as mentioned, and in addition about 20% protein and 70% predominantly complex carbohydrates.

Sound familiar? It should. That's essentially the diet recommended in my *Ripped* books and this column. The only real difference is that I allow a few ounces of lean meat or fish for flavoring, keeping fat to a minimum.

Mild Exercise Program

The experimental group was also asked to exercise (usually walking) for a minimum of three hours per week including 30 minutes per session at 50-80% of the individuals' age-adjusted maximum heart rate. In other words, they were put on a mild exercise program. Remember, these folks already had partially blocked coronary arteries. I suppose it would not have been a good idea to push them harder under the circumstances. Still, the results would probably have been even better had they been able to tolerate a more rigorous training program.

After a year the coronary arteries of all patients were again examined by computer-enhanced X-ray to determine what changes, if any, had occurred.

Ornish found that 82% of those on the very low fat diet showed an improvement in their heart's blood vessels. The average degree of clogging dropped from 61% to 56%. In the control group — get this — the degree of clogging *rose* from 62% to 64%. Importantly, patients in the experimental group reported a 91% drop in heart pain, generally within a few weeks. In contrast, control-group patients reported a 165% rise in heart pain frequency.

These changes in blockage may seem small, but they're actually very impressive when you consider that coronary blockage occurs over a period of decades. According to Ornish, one would not expect to find large changes in only one year. Plus, even a small amount of widening in clogged arteries has a large practical effect. This is demonstrated by the large reduction in heart pain in the experimental group as contrasted to the increased angina in the control group.

Remember too that even before the experiment both groups were already limiting their fat calories to 30% as recommended by the American Heart Association. Think about it. On a diet containing a relatively low 30% fat coronary artery blockage increased. Now, imagine what happens on the high-fat diet, 40% or more, most Americans consume.

Yes, this is big news. It proves for the first time that lifestyle changes alone — things you can do for yourself without the help of a doctor — may not only keep your coronary arteries clean and open but actually reverse blockage in only one year.

As you say, I once tried a high-protein (high protein almost always means high fat as well) low-carbohydrate diet. That was the diet many bodybuilders recommended a decade or so ago. In fact, Greg Ellis, Ph.D., in an interview by Editor-at-Large Jeff Everson in the May

1990 *Muscle & Fitness*, expressed the opinion that a high-fat, high-protein diet with only 20% carbohydrates will make your muscles grow faster. *Muscle & Fitness*, of course, didn't endorse that view, but simply presented Dr. Ellis' arguments for readers to evaluate.

In my books *Ripped* and *Ripped 2*, I explain at length why I soon abandoned the high-fat, low-carbohydrate diet. The main reason was that I felt tired and irritable. I couldn't think or train properly on that diet. Muscles need plenty of carbohydrates to function properly. Plus, fat makes you fat. And it has been known for a long time that fat, especially the saturated kind found in egg yolks, red meat and whole-milk products, contributes to coronary artery disease.

You ask about my blood lipid levels. My tests at the Cooper Clinic in 1988 and 1989 showed that my lifestyle does more than help me get ripped and stay that way. It probably prolongs my life. My laboratory evaluation showed that I had high normal to slightly elevated total cholesterol, LDL cholesterol (the bad kind) and triglyceride levels. Happily, it also showed that my HDL cholesterol (the good kind) is very high as a result of my regular exercise and very low bodyfat level. My total cholesterol/HDL ratio — the best indicator of coronary risk — is very good. Arno Jensen, my doctor at the Cooper Clinic, suspects that if I did not eat perfectly, maintain outstanding percent bodyfat and exercise that I would have very abnormal blood lipids. My father had to take medication to control his cholesterol, and Dr. Jensen believes that I have a genetic predisposition to have high cholesterol levels. So you see, my lifestyle does more than keep me lean. Dr. Jensen says it's critically important for my cardiovascular health.

I'll leave you with the common sense approach recommended by Lawrence E. Lamb, M.D., a frequent contributor to this magazine and editor of *The Health Letter*. To prevent heart disease follow three principles: "1) Stay lean, 2) Stay fit, 3) Don't smoke."

What's the best way to stay lean and fit? Why, the Ripped lifestyle, of course. It's the best bargain around: lean muscles and clean arteries.

PRIME SUSPECT

Inactivity is no longer just a secondary cause of heart disease

My mother — God rest her soul — used to say to me, with obvious annoyance, "You think exercise is the cure for everything!" Well, Mom, it looks like I was on the right track even as a know-it-all youngster. As I grow older and continue to exercise — and study — I become more and more convinced of the exercise/health connection.

I first learned of the relationship between exercise and health by reading *Strength & Health.* It made sense to me, even though I was mainly interested in developing some muscles to impress my classmates, that a strong, fit body would protect against disease. Decades later, I'm still an enthusiastic follower of the health-through-fitness doctrine.

The fundamental assumption that exercise will ward off disease has its roots in ancient Greek philosophy. The Greek ideal was a sound mind in a sound body, and the idea has gained credibility over the years.

Pioneers Of Health Through Exercise

William Blaikie & George Hackenschmidt led the way

Iron Game History, a publication edited by Terry and Jan Todd from the University of Texas at Austin, recently contained an article by Doug Bryant chronicling the work of William Blaikie, a late 19th-century American health reformer. A Harvard law school graduate, Blaikie, in 1883, published *How To Get Strong,* a book about the health benefits of regular exercise.

Blaikie was always interested in sports and physical fitness. At 17, he was lifting weights. In 1866, he was a member of the Harvard rowing crew that defeated Yale. For 10 years Blaikie held the amateur long-distance walking record, covering the 225 miles between Boston and New York in 4½ days. He helped found the Intercollegiate Athletic Games of America in 1873, one of the earliest collegiate track and field meets. He maintained an interest in physical education throughout his life, writing and lecturing frequently on the subject.

Blaikie believed sedentary living, which increased dramatically with the Industrial Age, was taking its toll on the health of Americans. His prescription: vigorous weight training, along with walking, running, rowing and swimming. Today, the notion that exercise can help prevent the onset of certain diseases is widely accepted.

That was not the case in Blaikie's time, however. In fact, one school of thought held that complete inactivity was the best way to prevent disease. For example, the accepted cure for neurasthenia, a common affliction of the day that we would probably characterize as stress disorder, was complete rest. *Iron Game History* describes the rest cure: "The patient was prescribed bed rest for a month or longer, was not allowed visitors or permitted to read or write, and was spoon-fed a diet of milk by a nurse."

Blaikie argued that the prevention — and cure — for neurasthenia was exercise. Like the ancient Greeks, he contended that a sound mind in a sound body is the recipe for success.

Another early advocate of exercise as a preventative was George Hackenschmidt, a turn-of-the-century strength athlete recently profiled by Terry Todd in *Iron Game History.* Known as the Russian Lion,

Hackenschmidt became the most famous wrestler in the world. After retirement, Hack, as he was called, became a philosopher and writer, lecturing at several of the best universities in the U.S. In 1909, Hackenschmidt published *The Way to Live,* a book setting forth his philosophy of health. "Apart from extraordinary causes, there is absolutely no reason why any man should ever be ill as long as he keeps his body so physically fit as to safeguard it against any breakdown," he wrote.

Hackenschmidt believed the lifestyle of his day left a man sickly. And, like Blaikie, his prescription was exercise. He believed in heavy weightlifting to increase strength, along with running and a diet of fresh foods. (How familiar that sounds!)

Lack of Exercise — As Dangerous As Smoking?

Exercise to prevent disease

Now, let's fast forward to the incident that triggered my look back at the old-timers who saw exercise as a prevention for disease. On July 1, 1992, the American Heart Association elevated physical inactivity or lack of exercise to the same level as cigarette smoking, high blood pressure and high cholesterol as a primary risk factor for coronary heart disease. (I hope you're listening, Mom.)

That's a momentous change. For years, inactivity was classified as a secondary risk. Says Kenneth H. Cooper, MD, founder of the Cooper Aerobics Center, whose scientists were primarily responsible for the underlying research, "Exercise has now been elevated to its proper place in the field of preventative cardiology." Wherever they are, Blaikie and Hackenschmidt must be smiling from ear to ear. I know I am.

Finally, Mom, here's a few lines from the Dec. 16, 1992 cover letter Arno L. Jensen, MD, enclosed with the report on my third and latest medical and fitness evaluation at the Cooper Aerobics Center in Dallas. "Clarence, once again your report is outstanding! Your overall health is superb. You practice the very best preventive medicine. I agree completely with your dietary and exercise advice. I recommend your books to many patients."

Importantly, Jensen warned that I have a natural tendency to develop elevated cholesterol and triglyceride levels, which increase my risk for heart disease. He also suspects that, like my dad, I am prone to develop adult-onset diabetes. Happily, Jensen believes that my diet and exercise habits help protect me from both ailments.

So, Mom, you can see why I still say, "Exercise is numero uno!"

CHAPTER TEN

THE AGE FACTOR

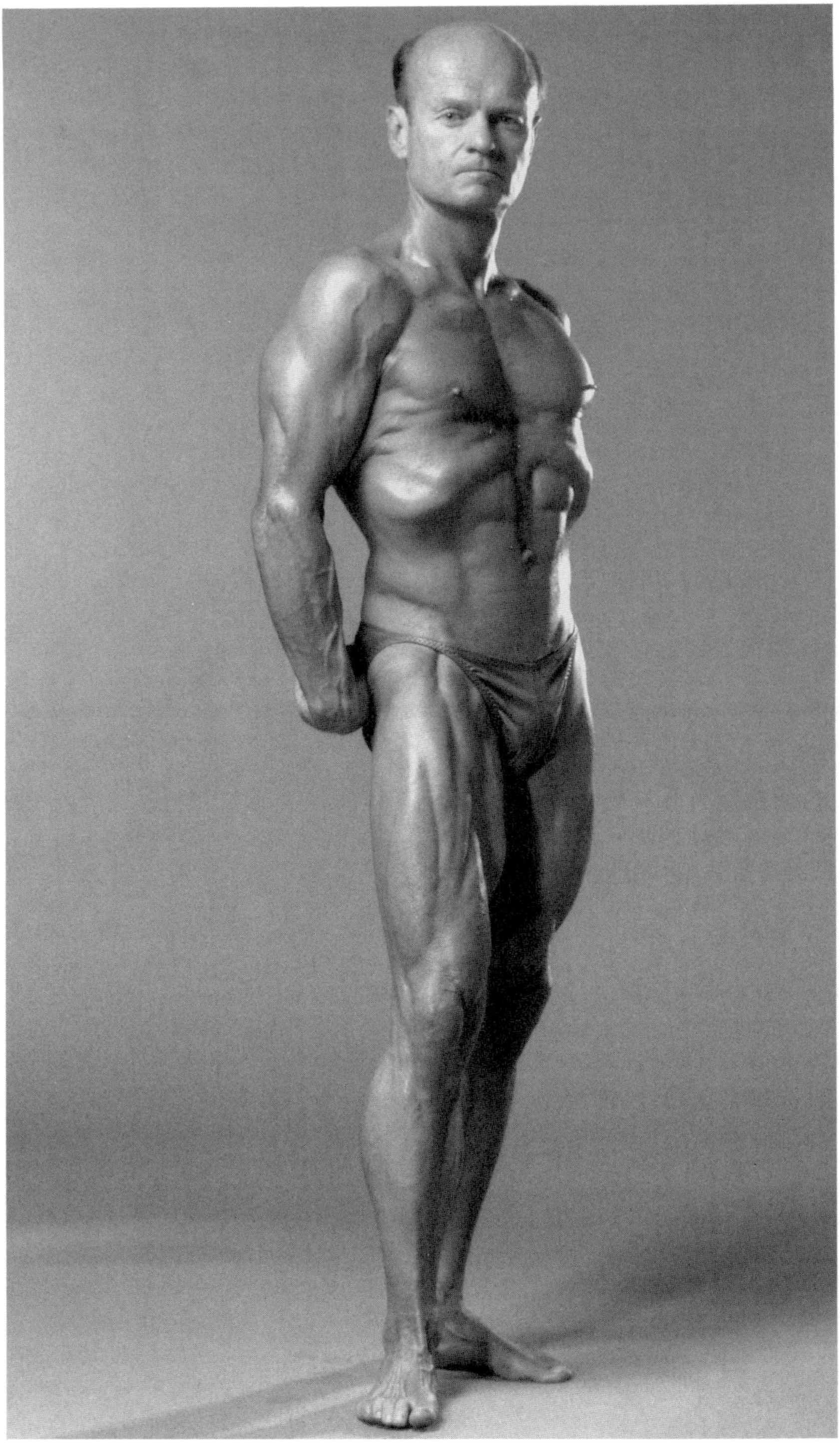

Another photo showing my condition at 55. *Photo by Pat Berrett.*

THE AGE FACTOR 10

STAY MOTIVATED

The day you stop exercising is the day you start aging

Q: *Several things happened to me recently that made me start to feel my age. First, I hurt my back changing a tire. I picked up a tire, and bam, had a spasm in my lower back. The pain and stiffness stayed with me for almost a month. Then I discovered that my foot was swollen and puffy. My doctor said I broke a blood vessel, a temporary condition that would soon clear up. It did.*

Finally, following close on these two rather ordinary problems, came a third symptom that's not really serious but bothered me emotionally. I had an erection and was amazed to see that my penis was bent. It looked like it had been in a wreck. I admit I laughed like hell, even though it was my *penis. The doctor again reassured me; it was simply a calcification in the tissues, which caused an uneven filling of the organ.*

All this put quite a strain on my self-image, but I'm back on an even emotional keel, thanks in great part to my steady progress in my weight training program.

A: Thanks for sharing the very personal indignities you've experienced recently. I'm pleased to hear that weight training is helping you weather the storm. The improvements you are making through bodybuilding obviously counterbalanced the curve balls nature and the aging process sent your way.

We're learning more every day about how exercise can slow or even reverse many of the physical and mental problems once blamed completely on aging. According to the *University of California, Berkeley Wellness Letter,* some experts estimate that half the functional losses that set in between ages 30 and 70 are in fact attributable to lack of exercise. "There is no drug in current or prospective use that holds as much promise for sustained health as a lifetime program of physical exercise," says the *Journal of the American Medical Association.*

Motivation Is The Problem

Exercise is the closest thing there is to the Fountain of Youth. That's clear. Motivation is the problem. How can we stay motivated to exercise for a lifetime? In his book *Ageless Athletes* (Contemporary Books, 1988) health psychologist and fitness expert Richard A. Winett addresses that question. He explores the motivational strategies of 17 of the most successful masters athletes, male and female, strength and endurance, including bodybuilders Bill Pearl, Frank Zane, Beverly Crown, Lynne Pirie and myself.

"Without exception," Winett states, "each athlete concurs that they are involved in a sport that ideally suits them temperamentally and genetically." In short, they found the activity that was right for them.

Some Eastern Bloc countries have massive testing programs to determine suitability for specific sports. In the West, we use mostly trial and error. That's what I did. In junior high school, I tried out for football. I made the team but soon decided I wasn't big enough. (I also didn't much like being tackled.)

My dad had been a champion in the high jump, broad jump, discus and pole vault. So I tried those events too. That didn't work either. First time out I dislocated my shoulder attempting to pole vault. Then I rolled out my father's barbell and tried weightlifting. That clicked almost immediately. It felt right. I liked the idea of an individual sport where you sink or swim based on your own individual efforts. Before I was out of high school, I won the city championship in Olympic lifting.

Obviously, everybody can't be a champion, and that's not necessary. The idea is to find an activity that appeals to you. Try an activity you enjoy, one that feels right.

You don't have to do the same thing for a lifetime, but you can if you wish. Most people change their emphasis or evolve in their sport or activity. I'll use my own example again, since that's what I know best. I focused mainly on the Olympic lifts until my middle 30s. By that time I was bumping up against my limits. I didn't think I could lift much more, and I really didn't feel motivated to try. So I switched to bodybuilding, where I could see myself improving a great deal. This brings me to Winett's second conclusion about motivation.

Success Breeds Success

All of Winett's ageless athletes set hard but reachable goals. Then they embarked on programs to achieve the goals they set for themselves. Mike Tymn, masters editor of *Runners' World* magazine and a four-time national masters champion himself, in a recent interview, said it perfectly: "As long as the person can continue to improve. he remains motivated."

That's basic. To stay motivated, you must find a goal, a realistic goal, that stimulates and excites you, and then you must make progress toward that goal. That's exactly what you are doing. Your goal, one that excites you, is to improve your body, through weight training. You're working to achieve that goal, and you're succeeding. This keeps you motivated. As I said in *Ripped 2,* "Success breeds success."

Finally, to help you stay motivated, here's another important message from *Ageless Athletes*: "In function and performance sense, the day you stop exercising and training is the day you start to age. And for those who are still sedentary, the day you start exercising and training is the day you begin to become younger!"

Stay motivated and you'll stay young.

CONCESSIONS TO AGE?

The main change is you need exercise — hard exercise — more

Q: *I would like to know how you had to adjust your workouts after reaching a certain age. A lot of us are aging and want to fight it.*

A: I'm not conscious of having made any adjustments in my workouts as a concession to age. Bodybuilding legend Bill Pearl, in a recent seminar, told the crowd he trains "virtually as hard as I ever did" — at 60. At 54, the same is true for me. Oh, sure, I have a few chronic injuries — a tender knee and a bad shoulder — which force some adjustments in how I do certain exercises. I always follow the time-honored rule: If it hurts, don't do it. But in terms of effort, my workouts haven't changed.

My interests have changed over the years, however. In my 30s, when I saw I wasn't going to improve as an Olympic lifter, I switched to bodybuilding, where I still had plenty of potential. At that time, I started using lighter weights and higher reps. (That gave my aging joints a new lease on life.) More recently, my interest has turned to balanced training; I now give equal emphasis to weights and aerobics. But again, through it all, I continued to train as hard as ever.

In fact, the main change that comes with age, as I see it, is that you need exercise — hard exercise — more. I discussed this last month. Perhaps this is a good time to tell you more about the increasing importance of exercise as we age.

Don't Give In

"Inactive people give aging a bad name," says noted cardiologist and fitness philosopher George Sheehan. What is usually perceived as aging, he explains, can be blamed largely on inactivity. Surprisingly,

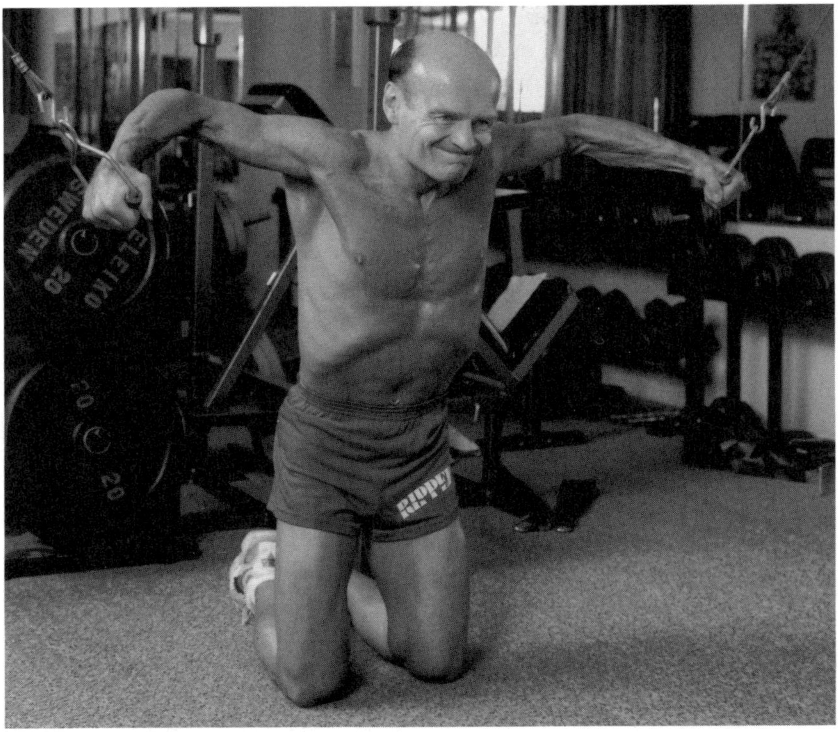

I appreciate the importance of exercise more with each year that goes by. *Photo by Pat Berrett.*

the average American is 30 years older functionally than he or she is chronologically. An active 60-year-old and an inactive 30-year-old will have equal physical work capacity. Sheehan says doctors who allow us to weigh more and have higher cholesterol because we've grown older do us no favor. In short, giving in to aging by becoming less active is a bad idea.

Dr. William Evans and Dr. Irwin Rosenberg, who wrote the landmark book *Biomarkers* (Simon & Schuster, 1991) discussed in my last column and who head up a team of scientists at the U.S. Department of Agriculture Human Nutrition Research Center on Aging at Tufts University, agree. According to them, the less physically active people become as they advance in years, the faster their bodies give out.

Evans and Rosenberg say, to stop the downhill slide that for many people begins at about 45, you need to push yourself physically. To fight the aging process effectively, you have to huff and puff and work up a sweat. You have to train hard. If that sounds inappropriate for someone in his or her 50s, 60s or even 70s or 80s, consider the example of my friend John North, a 65-year-old committed to the bodybuilding lifestyle.

North, in a recent letter, gleefully told me the reaction of "a neighbor kid in his late 30s" who saw him working outside with his shirt off. The neighbor shook his head as he stared at North's chest and slim middle. While claiming to be no match for some of the older bodybuilders he sees in *M&F,* North says, "compared to most men *half* my age, I'm like a young soldier at his peak of physical condition." To prove it, he does 50 push-ups straight and 150 in 15 minutes. Yes, like Bill Pearl and myself, North makes no concessions to age. He trains hard — and loves it.

Start Slowly

I don't mean to imply, of course, that older people who are new to exercise should plunge into hard training. That would be a mistake. Beginners and out-of-shape people — of any age — must ease into training gradually. "Start *slowly* and increase the vigor and duration of your activity as your fitness improves," advises the American Medical Association. Evans and Rosenberg advise such people to start out walking and then add weight training a few weeks later. What's more, the American College of Sports Medicine recommends that all men over 40 and all women over 50 have a medical exam before they begin vigorous training. This way you'll know if you have a condition that would limit your activity, such as heart disease, and also how intense your initial workouts should be. With clearance from your doctor and a period of break-in training under your belt, however, there's no reason to hold back on account of age.

According to Evans and Rosenberg, any healthy individual, regardless of age, should be able within a matter of 3-4 months to work up to a regimen of intense aerobic activity and weight training.

Don't Stop — Ever

Once you adjust to hard training, there's no reason to stop — ever. As a matter of fact, the more fitness you have, the more you stand to lose by slacking off. You need to keep training hard, because the beneficial effects of exercise are short-lived, they can't be "stored." Unfortunately, if you stop pushing, your condition starts to decline within one week.

"How old I look is important to me," says 70-plus George Sheehan. Me too. And that explains why I haven't lessened the intensity of my workouts as a concession to age. I want to look good — and feel good — as long as I can. To do that I know I have to keep straining, pushing my limits. Actually, I wouldn't have it any other way. Like John North, I love hard training. Nothing pays better dividends.

Here's the bottom line, from Evans and Rosenberg: "At any age, you're too old not to exercise."

HOW OLD IS OLD?

Age is a self-fulfilling prophecy

The caller's characterization of herself and her husband made my ears perk up. "We are senior citizens," she told the radio talk show host. "We're 58."

"Wait a minute," I thought. "Senior citizens — age 58?" The woman wanted to know how to invest a large retirement benefit her husband would soon receive so they could take it easy and travel.

To some, I suppose, that sounds like a dream come true, but I wonder. This woman is only a few years older than me, but her comments and tone of voice suggest that she thinks of herself and her husband as old. That could put a monkey wrench into their plans.

If you think you're old, you probably are. At one time 58 may have been considered old, but no more. As psychologist and social gerontologist Ken Dychtwald relates in *Age Wave* (Bantam Books, 1990), 58 is now considered young middle age. According to Dychtwald and Walter M. Bortz II, MD, author of *We Live Too Short and Die Too Long* (Bantam Books, 1991), true old age begins at 80. People are growing old much later than they used to, and the age of old age is likely to continue rising.

In 1900, 123,000 persons in America were over 85 years of age. Now there are three million. By 2050, Bortz estimates, 16% of the population or 50 million people in this country will be over 85. Tens of millions of people are living beyond age 65. In fact, the number of people who reached 65 during the past 100 years is equal to the number of those over age 65 who existed on this planet for all of history.

The Age Age

In their books, Dychtwald and Bortz convey the message that we are living a historic moment — a moment when a new, third age of life is appearing. Our time is commonly known as the Space Age, but Bortz says that it could just as well be called "the Age Age."

In the past there were only two ages, youth and adulthood. Youth ran from birth to around age 20, followed by adulthood, lasting from ages 20 to 65. Survivors past 65 were rare. Now, however, there are three segments of life: youth, from birth to around age 40; middle age, from 40-80; and old age, from 80-120.

Bortz, one of America's most respected authorities on aging, estimates that our biogenetic maximum lifespan is 120 years. No one should die until they are over 100, he contends. Any earlier deaths are premature. Bortz says, "As I recently passed my 60th birthday, halfway, it is like a golfer just starting the back nine."

Contrast the Bortz view with that of the lady on the radio. The difference, of course, is primarily attitude. "Age," says a 75-year-old quoted by Dychtwald, "isn't something on the calendar. It's just two things — your health and your attitude."

Fitness Guru

A good example is bodybuilding and fitness pioneer Jack LaLanne. At over 75, LaLanne still follows the routine he started half a century ago. He rises at 4:30 in the morning, and by 5 he's pumping iron. After two hours, he heads to the pool for an hour of swimming and water exercises.

When asked about retirement, he replies, "Retirement? No way! I don't care how long I live — I want to be 100% active and alive while I am living. Most Americans, hell, they die at 40, and they bury 'em at 70. Who wants that? I want to be productive. I want to be able to help people every day of my life!"

Now, that's the kind of attitude that keeps a person young!

Aging, Bortz tells us, is a self-fulfilling prophecy. Someone once observed, "Those who believe they *can't* are right; those who believe they *can* are right." When it comes to aging, we get what we expect.

Bortz cites many instances in which belief and health are intimately related. One of the best known is the placebo effect. Sugar pills work 10-20% of the time merely because of the strength of positive thinking. Persons intending suicide often die despite consuming sublethal doses of poison or despite having inflicted relatively trivial wounds.

Perhaps the most dramatic illustration of mind over matter concerns the ability of some practitioners of voodoo to cause others to die by suggestion. In one account: "In Australia, a witch doctor points a bone at a man. Believing that nothing can save him, the man rapidly sinks in spirits and prepares to die. He is saved only at the last minute when the witch doctor is forced to remove the charm."

Attitude Controls

Finally, Bortz describes an experiment at Johns Hopkins Medical School comparing the swimming endurance of wild and domesticated Norway rats. The researchers clipped the snout whiskers of the rats and then placed them in a swimming chamber. While a few of the tame rats died when put in the water, others swam for as long as 81 hours. Every one of the 34 wild rats, however, immediately sank to the bottom of the tank and died. Apparently the wild rats perished not because their whiskers were clipped, but they seemed to give up because they were held. (Veterinarians call this "capture myopathy," a condition where a pursued animal topples over and dies with no apparent injury.) The tame rats, of course, were accustomed to being held.

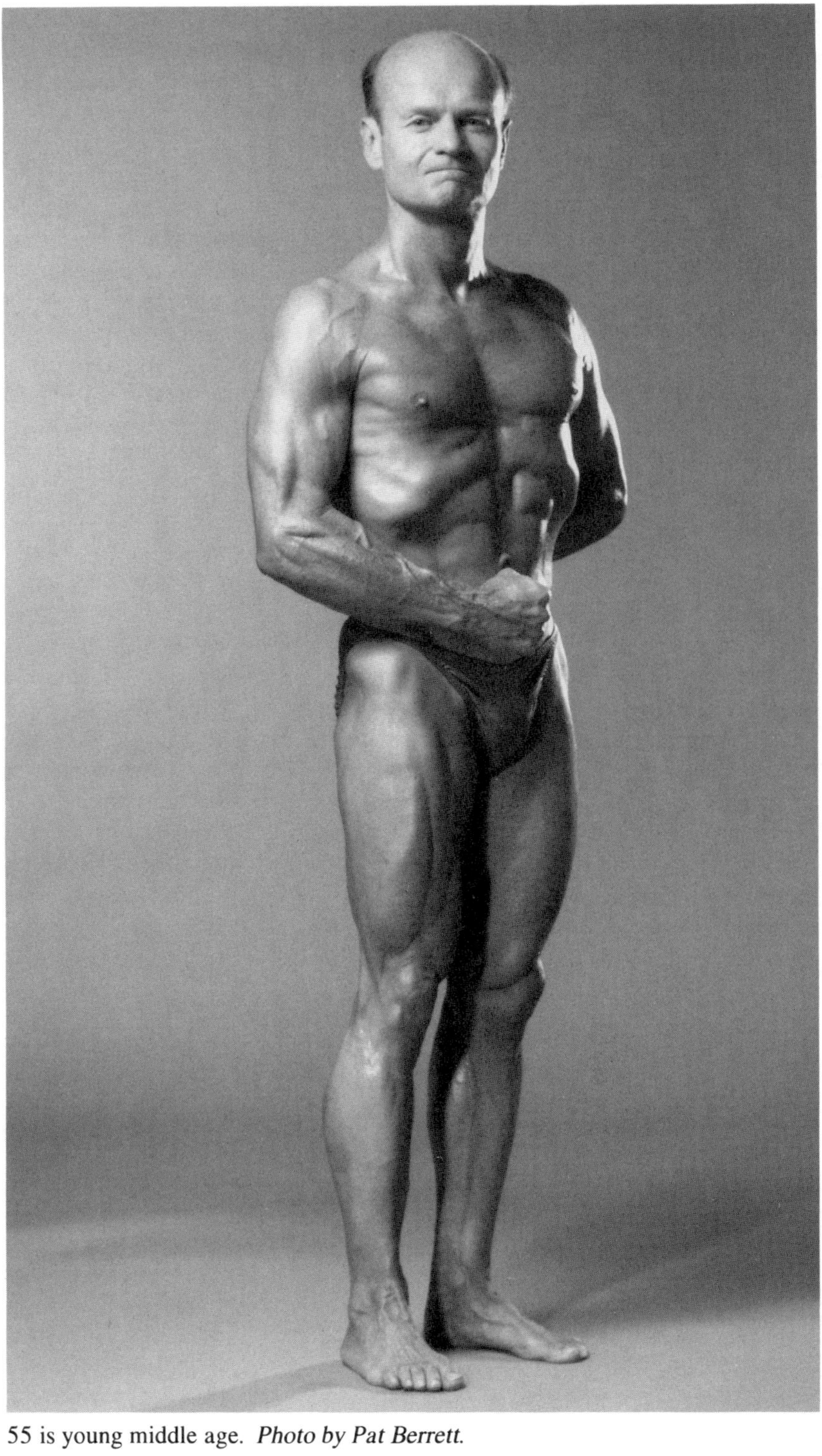

55 is young middle age. *Photo by Pat Berrett.*

In subsequent experiments the rats first were held and then released; next they were immersed in water for just a few seconds, then rescued. The result was that the wild rats *learned* not to give up. They swam as long as their domesticated cousins. Again, attitude was the controlling factor.

In short, we tend to do and become what we expect to do and become. If we decide that we are old, then we are old. "The accuracy of your prediction is guaranteed," says Bortz, "because of the attitudes, decisions and health habits conspiring to assure their own fulfillment." What was once thought to be aging, we can now confidently attribute to disease and, more importantly, disuse. Pneumonia, tuberculosis and other life-shortening diseases have for the most part been conquered. For the first time in history, we have the opportunity to live out our full 100-120 year lifespan. The only things that stand in the way are our attitudes and lifestyles.

Seven Rules

Here are seven rules for a long and healthy life from George Sheehan, MD:

1) Exercise regularly.
2) Eat a good breakfast.
3) Don't eat between meals.
4) Maintain optimal weight (usually your weight at age 25).
5) Don't smoke.
6) Drink moderately (or not at all).
7) Get a good night's sleep.

Such simple rules. Let's follow them — and not talk ourselves into premature old age. We fulfill our own prophecies. It's up to us — to you —to decide.

THE COMPETITIVE EDGE

The will to win makes for a longer, more robust life

A revolution is taking place in our understanding of the aging process. Most people take it for granted that aging means an inevitable physical decline. For years, medical scientists have said that after 25 we lose about 1% per year in aerobic capacity (VO_2 Max), strength, speed and a whole host of physical attributes. That's just the way it is, gerontologists have maintained. Well, it's now becoming increasingly clear that it doesn't have to be that way. In fact, the 1%-per-year rule of thumb may have little, if any, application to individuals who continue to train at a competitive level.

In past columns I've mentioned Dr. Michael Pollock's study of 24 healthy, active men who continued to train after the normal competitive period. At the beginning of the study in 1971, all were 40 or over and considered champion Master athletes, mostly runners. Ten years later, when Pollock tested the men again, he found that those who had continued to train hard showed much less deterioration from aging. Surprisingly, at least to adherents of the old rule of thumb, the men who continued to train for high-level competition maintained their ability to consume oxygen; over the 10-year period of the study, their VO_2 Max barely declined. Those who allowed training intensity to drop off, however, showed a marked decline over the same period; their VO_2 Max declined by an average of 12.5%, compared to a decline of only 1.7% for the competitive group.

With every year that goes by, support continues to build for Pollock's finding that the key to holding off the aging process is hard training. For example, my friend Richard Winett, Ph.D., a professor of psychology at Virginia Tech in Blacksburg and author of the *Master Trainer* newsletter, recently called my attention to a highly encouraging study of male competitive swimmers over a 15-year span.

"For scientists studying the aging process, Masters swimming provides a natural laboratory with tens of thousands of subjects," wrote Phil Whitten, Ph.D., in the July/August 1992 issue of *Swim.* Master's swimming involves athletes more than 20 years old and provides precise performance data on competitors in 5-year age brackets, from 25-75. This allowed Whitten to study the same individuals over an extended period. He compared the best times in four different age groups every five years. For example, Group A was 25-29 in 1975, 30-34 in 1980, 35-39 in 1985, and 40-44 in 1990. Thus he was able to measure how performances changed over 15 years.

"Dramatic Finding"
Swimming delays decline

Here's a summary of the exciting results: For men who swim regularly, physical decline begins not at 25, but in the mid-30s. In fact, these men are actually faster in their early 30s than in their late 20s. Decline begins almost imperceptibly for these swimmers. They do not decline at the 1%-per-year rate until they reach their early 70s.

"This is a dramatic finding," says Whitten. It means that the 1%-decline-per-year-after-age-25 rule applies only to those who lead a sedentary lifestyle; they lose 25% of their physical capacity by the age of 50 and by 75 they have lost 50%.

In contrast, if you swim regularly — and competitively — the decline is only 3.5% by the age of 50 and 19.1% by 75. Another way to look at it is a 70-year-old competitive swimmer will have the strength and vitality of a "normal" 45-year-old.

What's more, Whitten believes that his results actually understate what is theoretically possible. "Almost all of the decline, I believe, is due to a sedentary, unhealthy lifestyle." Most Masters swimmers have families and job responsibilities, Whitten observed. They are unable to train more than an hour or so a day. "Were they able to put in the time and mileage top collegiate swimmers do, they probably could swim even faster."

Like Pollock, Whitten believes the secret to maintaining performance with advancing age is to never let yourself get out of condition. He speculates that the much-publicized comeback attempt by swimmer Mark Spitz failed not because of age, but because Spitz took a 16-year break from training after his seven-gold-medal performance at the 1972 Olympics. Whitten calculates, based on his study of Masters swimmers, that a 42-year-old Spitz would have been capable of swimming .05 of a second faster than his world record 20 years earlier — "if he'd never stopped [swimming] at all after Munich."

As it turned out that time would have placed Spitz third at the Olympic trials. That doesn't seem at all far-fetched, when you consider that 37-year-old Lorraine Moller of New Zealand placed third in the women's marathon at Barcelona, only a little more than a minute behind the winner. And don't forget that Francie Larrieu-Smith, the top American finisher, was 39.

My own years of regular, hard training — weights and aerobics — have produced results consistent with Whitten's findings. My aerobic fitness has been tested twice at the Cooper Clinic, first in 1988 when I was almost 51 and again a year later. My first test produced a treadmill time of 28 minutes, placing me better than 1½ minutes above the 99th percentile for the 50-59 age group. In 1989 my treadmill time improved to 29 minutes. My goal next time, when I'm 55, is 30 minutes. So you see, I can testify firsthand that decline with age is not inevitable.

CHAPTER ELEVEN

THE LEAN LIFESTYLE

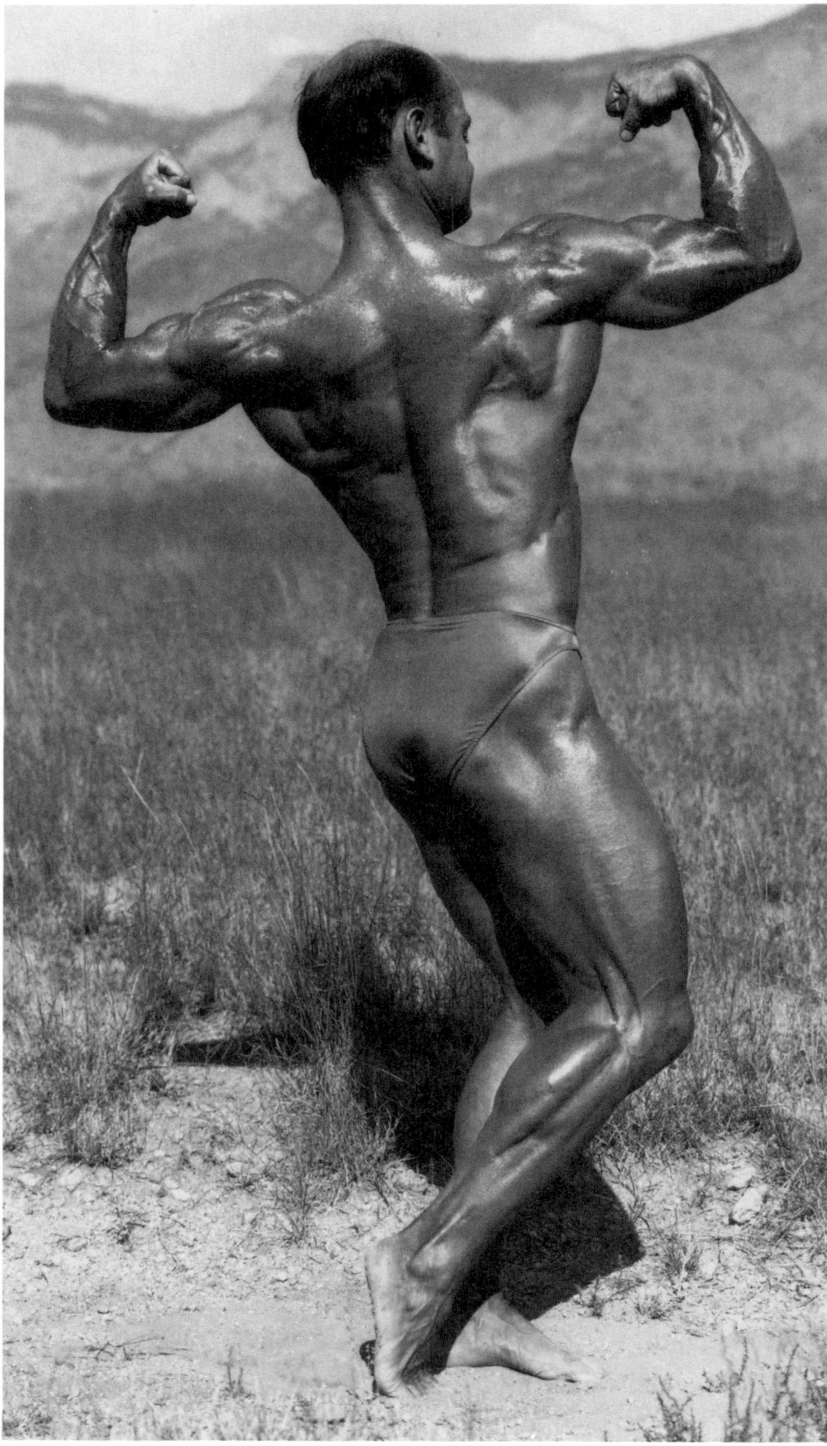

Photo by Guy Appelman.

THE LEAN LIFESTYLE 11

FRESH STARTS

Make fitness a permanent part of your life

Q: *I've been an insurance claims man for 38 years, the last 20 deskbound as a litigation specialist. I've been an exercise freak for 10 years now, but only recently discovered weight training. I feel like I'm into a challenging new career — bodybuilding. There will be dog days of struggle, but I'm really excited about getting leaner and stronger. I know your books and* Muscle & Fitness *will help.*

A: Congratulations! You've discovered the way to beat the boredom that causes so many people to fall off the exercise wagon. You've found a new mountain to climb, so to speak, one that challenges and excites you, and on which you can realistically expect to make progress.

A recent headline in *The Wall Street Journal* read: "The Exercise Boom Loses Its Strength." Exercise is out, the article said. "The couch potato is more popular than the marathoner today," a fitness and management consultant complained.

The same issue of *The Journal* reported that a thriving business had sprung up in the purchase and sale of used fitness equipment. Sports Consignment Center, a Houston shop, "buys from the dispirited and sells to the optimistic, sometimes recycling the same stuff over and over." Apparently, such shops are cropping up around the country. They're all based on the premise that more than half the people who start exercise programs drop out within six months.

Why so many dropouts? A 24-year-old fitness fanatic who swam, lifted weights and rode an exercise bike told *The Journal* why he quit: "Boredom." He'd simply had his fill of working out. That's probably the main reason why most people quit — the particular activity no longer challenges and excites them.

Three Examples

Far fewer would drop out, I'm convinced, if, when progress stops or interest wanes, they would make a fresh start, like you're doing. Exercise can be a permanent part of your life if you constantly seek out stimulating new goals — realistic, achievable goals suited to your stage of development. Let me give you three examples — a reigning Olympic champion, an aging athlete still in shape, and myself.

Louise Ritter

After 15 years, Louise Ritter achieved her dream in Seoul. She won the Olympic gold medal for the high jump. Still, as Kenny Moore wrote in *Sports Illustrated,* after returning home to Dallas, Ritter went through a period of despondency. "I couldn't figure out what was wrong," she said. "Everything I wanted happened, and I'm depressed?" Why? Moore explained: "Because a goal achieved is a goal lost." Obviously, she needed a new goal, a fresh start.

Ritter, who incidentally helped start a Dallas company that sells used sporting equipment, has worked through her despair. She's now back in hard training with a new goal. She's aiming for a new world record.

Here's how it happened. High-speed film taken at the US Olympic trials last summer shows that she cleared 6′6¼″ by enough to put her easily over a world record 6′11″. Reviewing that film made her realize that on a good day under the right conditions she's capable of establishing a new world record. Presto! The clouds lifted. No more depression. She has an exciting, and for her realistic, new challenge. Like you, she has a fresh start.

George Sheehan, M.D.

George Sheehan, MD, running's top guru, told recently in *The Physician and Sportsmedicine* how a switch to biking gave him a "new beginning." Sheehan, now in his 70s and suffering from prostate cancer, was losing his competence in running, and with it the enjoyment. "Not only do I now have difficulty running," he wrote, "but I also remember when I was good at it. That is the worst part — knowing that it may never be the way it was."

For Sheehan, the bike was different. Like your bodybuilding, with cycling he was starting a new career, one where he could improve without looking back on the former excellence he could never again achieve. As he put it: "When I run, I am an old man. When I bike, I am a child again... My body thinks it is good at cycling and getting better." In cycling, Sheehan found a new joy in exercise, or in his words, "a new addiction."

You can find the same thing in bodybuilding. I did.

Clarence Bass

In 1976, at 39, I was at a crossroads. I had been a good Olympic

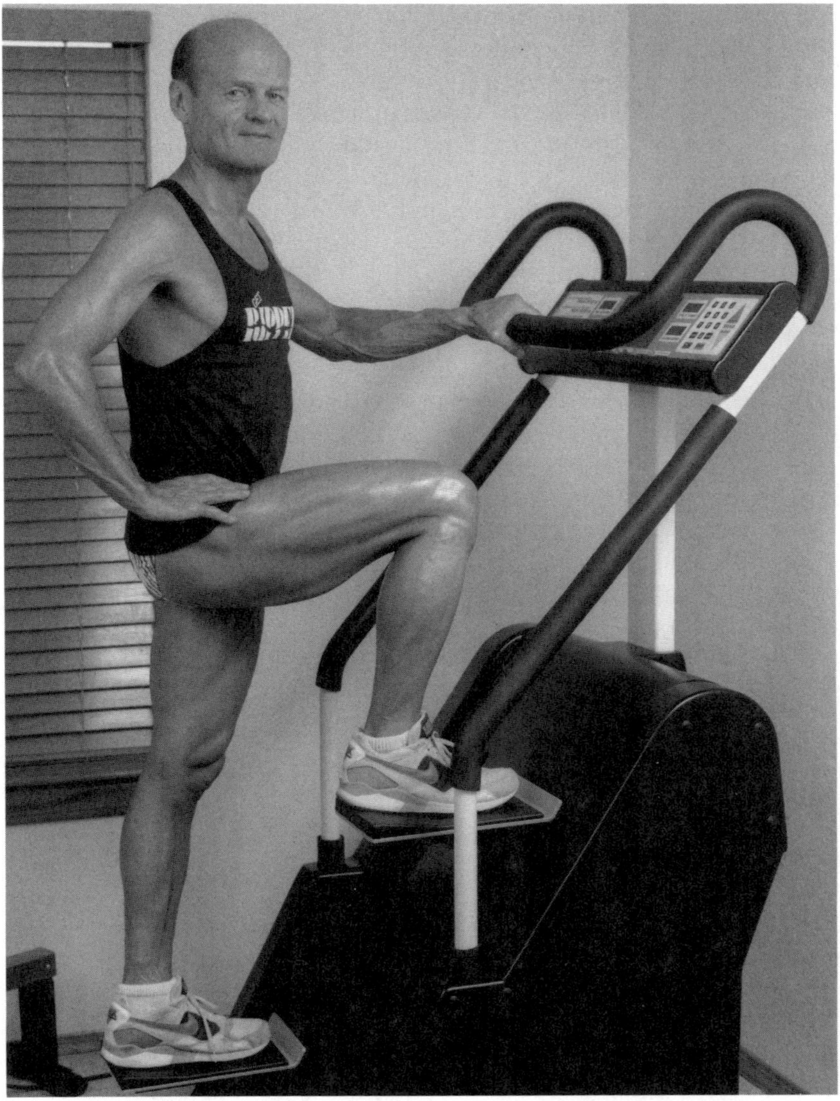

I'm always looking for new mountains to climb. *Photo by Pat Berrett.*

lifter and a respectable powerlifter as well, but it was clear I wasn't going to get any better. In those sports, my best days were behind me. That's when I saw Vic Seipke win the Past 40 Mr. America title and decided to enter bodybuilding competition myself. I had seen Vic win the 1955 Junior Mr. America when I competed in the Junior National Olympic Lift Championship, and I was one of the judges at the 1976 Past 40 Mr. America competition, where Vic became the first National Masters physique champion. As I wrote in *Ripped,* "I was thrilled to see Vic looking as good in 1976 as he did in 1955."

Inspired by Seipke's success, I decided that I, too, could be a

National Masters physique champion. As you probably know, that's what I did. In short, bodybuilding gave me a tremendous new enthusiasm for exercise. It gave me a fresh start.

Now at 51, I still use the fresh start principle to maintain my enthusiasm for staying lean and fit. I'm constantly on the lookout for new mountains to climb.

As you know from reading my column, last year my challenge was to do well on the treadmill test at the Cooper Clinic. I literally climbed a mountain, one near my house, training to achieve that goal. Like the treadmill, the mountain starts easy and gradually gets steeper and steeper. It turned out to be a perfect proxy for the Cooper Clinic test. My treadmill time of 28 minutes placed me in the top category for men under 30, and 1½ minutes above the 99th percentile for men my age.

As I write this, I'm training hard on the Concept II rower in preparation for submitting my 2,500-meter time for placement on the world ranking list published annually by Concept II, Inc. When that's done, I'll begin preparing for a rematch with the treadmill. I'm shooting for a time of 30 minutes when I go back to the Cooper Clinic in the fall for retesting. That's a realistic goal for me. My heart beats faster just thinking about it.

The bottom line is this: continually search for exercise goals that challenge and excite you. Train for and achieve your goal, and then formulate another. That way, you'll never be bored, and you'll never become an exercise dropout.

WHEN YOUR BODY COMPLAINS

In training, as in life, you have to back off and change course occasionally

A recent caller to Ripped Enterprises told my wife Carol that he considers me a "living experiment." It doesn't seem possible, not to me anyway, but my one-man experiment has been going on now for 40 years. That's how long I've been training. I started lifting when I was 13, and I'm still going strong at 53.

A few days ago, I read a story in the *Washington Post* about boxer Sugar Ray Leonard, who was preparing to fight Terry Norris for the World Boxing Council's junior-middleweight title. I read it with special interest, because in a way it captured the essence of why my experiment has been successful for so long. The piece questioned why Leonard was still fighting at 34. He's won five world titles and has plenty of money. He could be embarrassed or, worse, permanently injured. Why does he go on fighting?

Leonard's answer was simple and to the point: "This is what I enjoy."

Well, as you probably know, Leonard lost a 12-round decision. "It definitely is my last fight," Leonard said. The follow-up story added, "Leonard isn't an old man, but on this night before 7,495 fans, he sure was an old fighter."

I won't be surprised if Leonard changes his mind — how many times would that be? — and signs for a rematch with Norris. That's not my point, however. The message is in what Sugar Ray said before and after the fight.

"This is what I enjoy," Leonard said. That's true for me as well with training. Training has been my most reliable source of success. I understand it. I control it. It works. So I keep doing it.

Leonard changed his tune after the fight. "My son (17-year-old Ray Jr.) told me I was an old man," said Leonard. "Maybe he was right."

Backing Off

In short, Leonard decided to cool it, at least for the time being. I too have backed off a number of times during my training career. In fact, having the flexibility to back off or change course from time to time is, in large part, responsible for my training longevity.

In *Ripped 2,* I explained how the hard-day, easy-day training concept pioneered by track coach Bill Bowerman at the University of Oregon can help bodybuilders make better gains. Runners, like bodybuilders, once thought they had to train hard every day, but Bowerman said that every hard day should be followed by one, two, three or more easy days, until the body is recovered and ready for another hard session.

Hal Higdon, a worldclass runner now in his 60s, explained recently in *Runner's World* that Bowerman's hard/easy philosophy applies in a broader sense as well, over a lifetime. "Hard weeks can be followed by easy weeks, hard months by easy months, hard years by easy years, hard decades by easy decades," he wrote.

Higdon speaks from experience. Starting in high school, he's been running all his life. Importantly, however, not all his running has been hard. He didn't really mature as a runner until after college, reaching worldclass status in his late 20s. Then he spent a long period away from serious running "until the Masters movement came along and collected me." His return to peak condition produced a Masters world championship. More recently, he spent a decade "playing around with other sports such as skiing and cycling." He's now running hard again, focusing on the World's Veterans Championships this summer in Turku, Finland.

Through it all, Higdon says he's learned one important lesson: "When training through the seasons of your life, you don't always need to run at your peak. You don't need to struggle to be in top shape all the time... You can let yourself relax, then get excited about running again."

My training career has followed a similar pattern. I spent my teen years and my 20s as a competitive Olympic lifter. During my 30s I continued to train, but with less intensity as I devoted my major efforts to the practice of law. Then, like Higdon, my training intensified again under the stimulation of over-40 competition. After winning my class in National Masters Bodybuilding Competition, I continued to lift, but with more of an emphasis on fitness and endurance, and competing mainly with myself.

Lifetime Training

I'll wrap this up with three recent examples of my approach to lifetime training: one case where I backed off, one where I didn't, and another where I should have.

My first test on the Cooper Clinic treadmill in 1988 was an exciting new challenge. I'd read Dr. Kenneth Cooper's classic *Aerobics* shortly after it was published in 1968 and, from time to time, had seen reports on famous athletes who'd been tested at his clinic. So when Dr. Arno Jensen invited me to come to Dallas for testing, I jumped at the opportunity. I'd never been on a treadmill and didn't know how I'd do. But Jensen assured me that my training combination, weights and aerobics, was good preparation. I lasted 28 minutes, which placed me well above the 99th percentile for my age group.

The next year was different. I tossed and turned in my bed at the Aerobics Center guest lodge the night before my rematch with the treadmill. All I could think about was the distress and pain that was coming. As David Prokop later wrote in *Muscle & Fitness,* "A treadmill test to exhaustion is a journey to nowhere in which the destination isn't a place, but a physical state [of total fatigue]." I exceeded my previous year's time by a full minute, but it was not fun, believe me.

Obviously, it was time to back off. After returning home I wrote Jensen that I wouldn't be back the next year.

A New Challenge

I needed a new goal. I found it in indoor rowing competition, which simulates rowing on the water, using a machine made by Concept II, Inc.

At that time I'd been rowing for about two years and had placed in the middle third of the Concept II company's 1989 world ranking for men aged 50-59. I decided to challenge myself by entering a competition to be held in Denver early in 1990. It was a good experience. I set a new personal record and came home inspired to train at a faster pace, and then try to move up in the world ranking. That's what I did. I improved on my 2,500-meter time in Denver by almost 15 seconds, which moved me into the upper 25% for lightweights in the 1990 ranking. I wrote in my diary: "A great effort, but I don't want to do that again anytime soon."

In training for competition and then the personal record attempt, I'd developed quite an aversion to rowing 2,500 meters (a little over 1½ miles). "The event is comparable to running a 440-yard dash for two miles," a coach at the 1990 World Indoor Rowing Championships told *The Wall Street Journal.* "A normal body shouldn't be put under such strain," she added.

So I faced a hard decision when the entry blank came for the rowing competition this year. I don't think I'd have entered if the Rocky Mountain Rowing Club hadn't developed a new condensed format for 1991. The previous year, I especially disliked the idea of rowing 2,500 meters twice, once in the preliminaries and again in the finals. One hard 2,500-meter piece is plenty. Happily, the format called for all finals, no heats.

I couldn't resist. I decided to go for it again; and I'm glad I did. I improved my time by nine seconds and moved up from seventh in 1990 to second this year. It was another good experience.

As I write this I'm training for a new personal record to send in for the 1991 Concept II world ranking. In short, I'm still feeling good about rowing. It's one of the hardest things I've ever done. Nevertheless, at this point anyway, the satisfaction I get from continued improvement makes it worthwhile.

A Lesson Learned

Finally, like Sugar Ray Leonard, I recently went for it one time too many. I violated a time-honored rule: if it hurts, don't do it. Now I'm paying for it.

Years ago, I injured my left shoulder doing an overhead lift. I've had to guard it ever since. It acted up again last year as I prepared for my Joe Weider photo session. In particular, the shoulder hurt doing curls. I tried to be careful, but I foolishly kept curling.

When I returned home I kept curling. Well, a few days ago my luck ran out. I heard a big pop. I knew something had happened, but strangely I had no pain. In fact, the discomfort I had in my shoulder disappeared.

Later, however, I observed an enlargement in my left biceps. I had partially detached the short head from its origin in the shoulder area. My doctor says it will reattach in its new location; if I'm lucky the only aftereffect will be a new peak in my left biceps. I'm not supposed to do anything strenuous with the arm until it's fully healed. (Fortunately, rowing doesn't hurt the injured area.)

The lesson is pretty clear: when your body complains, pay attention.

YOU'VE GOT THE POWER

Q: *Six months ago my doctor informed me that my LDL cholesterol (the bad kind) was high, and I went nuts. I've always prided myself on being active and never had health problems. I read your books cover to cover and immediately went on a low-fat, high-fiber diet and started working out extra hard. My doctor now says my HDL cholesterol (the good kind) is extremely high and that my LDL cholesterol has returned to an acceptable level. You've rejuvenated my interest. I now recommend your books to all my friends who are just waking up to the significance of diet combined with exercise.*

A: Congratulations! With a little prodding from your doctor, you've taken control of your body. That's good news indeed, with more far-reaching ramifications than you may realize.

If you break your leg, get busted up in a car wreck or need your appendix removed, your doctor can help. However, when you step out of the realm of crisis intervention into the multitude of ailments that sneak up over the course of a lifetime and refuse to go away — diseases related to lifestyle such as diabetes, high blood pressure, osteoporosis, clogged coronary arteries and ulcers — I believe your doctor will agree that you can do far more for yourself than he or she can. In the final analysis, you — and only you — are responsible for your health on an ongoing basis. You're the engineer in charge, so to speak. That's where diet, exercise and stress management come to the fore.

It's wonderful to realize, as you have recently, that you can do something — a lot, really — to help yourself. Actually, lifestyle change, something almost completely in your hands, can take you from a condition of simply being free from illness — your doctor's area of expertise — to a state of superhealth. That, to use the buzzword of the '90s, is "empowerment."

As I say, the beneficial effects of taking control of your body and your life are far-reaching. Studies at Yale, Harvard and elsewhere have shown that the greatest risks for illness occur when people have little control over their lives. That's also when they experience the most stress.

According to preventative medicine specialists Neil F. Gordon, MD and Larry W. Gibbons, MD, authors of *The Cooper Clinic Cardiac Rehabilitation Program* (Simon & Schuster, 1990), excessive stress over an extended period can weaken the body's immune systems. We become less able to ward off sickness.

The feeling of helplessness — that you're no longer in charge, either of an event or of yourself — is one of the classic stressors. To illustrate the connection between control and stress, Gordon and Gibbons ask us to picture a two-person bobsled team hurtling down a hill. "Who has

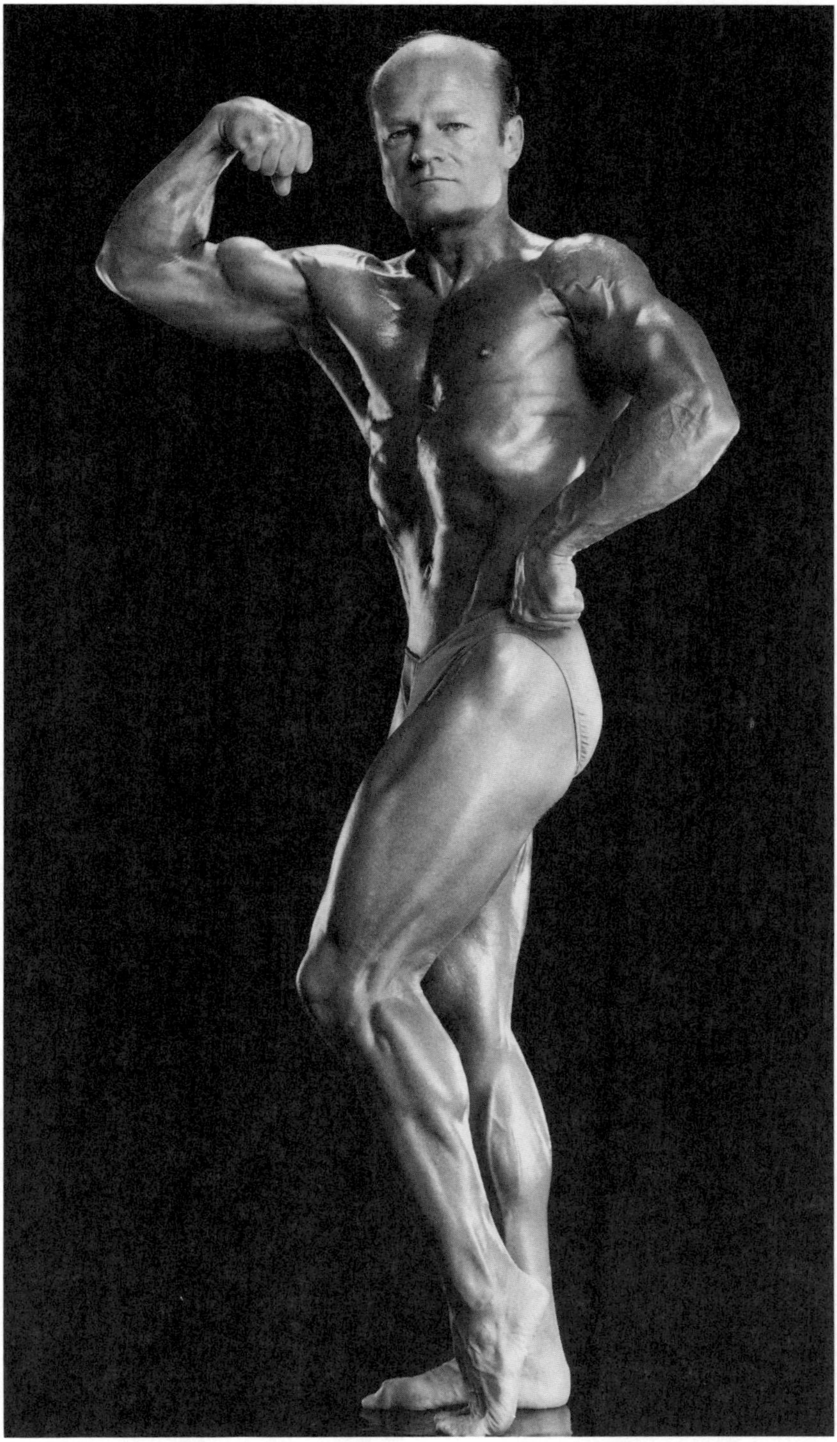

Photo by John Balik.

the most stress," they ask, "the person in the front who is driving, or the one in the back who's along for the ride?" The person in the back, of course, because that individual has no control.

Channeling Stress

Stress per se, of course, is not the problem. Stress is inevitable. We all experience stress. Some stress, in fact, is desirable. Many of our most rewarding experiences represent examples of stress channeled to highly productive ends. The problem comes when stress gets out of hand and our bodies produce too much of the high-voltage "fight or flight" chemicals that, among other things, speed up our heart rate and raise our blood pressure. In other words, the problem is not stress in and of itself, but how we react to it. That's another area where regular exercise helps.

Dr. Kenneth H. Cooper, the founder of the world-renowned Cooper Clinic in Dallas, called exercise "nature's tranquilizer." It's practically impossible to feel stress when you're pleasantly pooped after an exercise session. Every athlete — bodybuilders and others — knows that sense of relaxation and well-being that comes after a good workout. Cooper and others believe that exercise triggers the release of endorphins, hormones that produce a sense of euphoria — a feeling that all is right with the world. Once endorphins enter the bloodstream, their beneficial effects are thought to last two or three hours. There's more to it than that, however.

As noted earlier, when people lose control they feel stressed, as you did when your doctor dropped the bombshell about your LDL cholesterol. Regular exercise (and a low-fat diet) restored your equilibrium. Six months later, when you learned that your good cholesterol was up and your bad cholesterol down, you experienced a sense of self-reliance and self-esteem. You were back in the driver's seat. And that may be even more important to your health than your cholesterol level.

Furthermore, the sense of self-mastery that came with your victory over your cholesterol level will carry over into all parts of your life. The sense of confidence and control you found through diet and exercise will not only make you healthier and more resistant to disease, it will help you react more positively to everything you encounter in life.

I expressed essentially the same thought in *Ripped 2* when I wrote: "The hour or so I spend in my gym calms me for the rest of my day. Controlling the stress I undergo in my gym fortifies me for the chaos on the outside." And today, I'm more convinced than ever that it's true. Bodybuilding, you see, helps me in everything I do.

THE PLAINS TRUTH

To bring out your best, get primitive!

Q: *I am a man, 43, 6′5″ and 300 pounds. I used to be extremely active. I played football and basketball and lifted weights. But in the last 15 years I've gained a lot of fat and lost a lot of muscle tone. Now I want to get fit and ripped for the rest of my life. You have inspired me to start exercising again, and any advice to help me stay motivated would be greatly appreciated.*

A: Congratulations! Walter M. Bortz II, MD, author of *We Live Too Short and Die Too Long* (Bantam Books, 1991), would say that you have decided to return to the ways of our evolutionary ancestors. That's good news indeed.

Bortz, one of America's most respected and acclaimed authorities on aging, has for years explored the effects of inactivity on the functioning of the human body. His study of disuse goes back millions of years to the time when our ancestors first walked upright on two legs, and left the jungle and went out onto the plain. We know from footprints found by anthropologist Mary Leakey in Tanzania that this occurred at least 3.76 million years ago.

Bortz says that this was a historic event in the evolution of mankind; whereas food in the jungle was near at hand, on the plains things were different. Only the fittest survived. On the savannas early man was forced to run down his prey; he also had to be strong enough to carry it back to camp.

Primitive humans, when compared to other predators, were at a competitive disadvantage. They were small, slow and had no claws or killing jaws and teeth like the large cats. So what was it that allowed man to survive? Bortz says it was his ability to run long distances: "The human endurance capacity is virtually unique."

The big cats give up the chase if unsuccessful after a quarter mile or so, but early man had the capacity to run down the plains animals (mostly antelope) simply by the strategy of keeping them constantly on the run in the midday sun until they were completely exhausted and could be easily killed.

"Zoo Animals"

Our hunter-gatherer era lasted until the Agricultural Revolution, which occurred some 10,000 years ago. Until that time, Bortz says, we lived our lives in an extraordinarily active mode. "The food moved and we moved." After the Agricultural Revolution, however, we no longer chased our food; we grew it. And, of course, with the arrival of the Industrial Revolution just 200 years ago, we stopped chasing or cultivating our food and simply bought it at the store. In the words of Bortz,

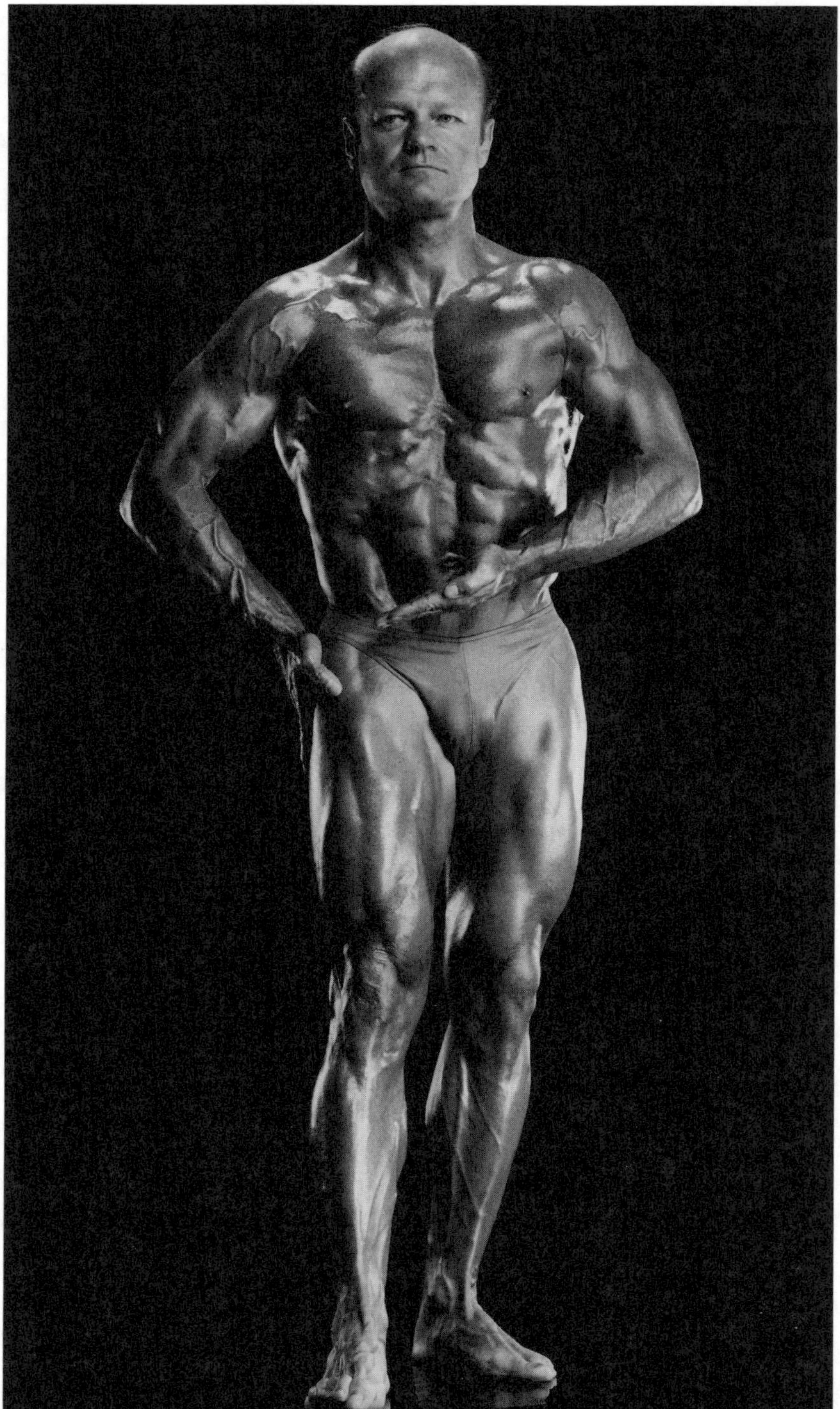

Photo by John Balik.

"We became zoo animals."

You know what happens to animals when they are confined and supplied with regular food without being required to exert themselves to find it or run it down. They get fat and lose muscle tone — just like you have in the last 15 years.

To illustrate how unnatural is the inactive lifestyle of modern man, Bortz uses Carl Sagan's convention of conforming a given time span to a calendar year. If we set the morning of January 1 as 3.76 million years ago, the time when we know we were upright, 200,000 generations of man lived the vigorous life of the hunter-gatherer, until the Agricultural Revolution occurred early on the morning of December 31. Significantly, on that time scale the Industrial Revolution arrived only in the final second of the year, at 11:59:59 p.m.

"The conclusion," writes Bortz, "is that throughout the long span of our prehistory, our evolutionary development, we lived as physically active, vigorous creatures of robust vitality." In other words, our bodies are made to run long and lift heavy. We are simply not suited for the inactivity of the modern world.

By deciding to become active again you have, in effect, returned to your roots. You have decided to live the active life for which your body was designed. You have decided to strive for true normalcy and give up the modern lifestyle, the lifestyle symbolized by the motorized golf cart.

"It is my feeling," says Bortz, "that if we were asked to embalm one item in a time capsule which would serve to tell generations 10,000 years from now who we, as a culture, were, the best choice would be the golf cart. It tells our story eloquently."

Like the automobile, the electric carving knife, escalators and elevators, the golf cart shows just how far we have departed from our evolutionary past.

Fitness philosopher and cardiologist George Sheehan supports Bortz's conclusions that the inactive lifestyle is, in fact, abnormal. The average American, according to Sheehan, is 30 years older functionally than he or she is chronologically. An active 60-year-old and an inactive 30-year-old will have equal physical work capacity.

Again, Sheehan believes, this can be blamed largely on inactivity. Displaying his famous dry wit, Sheehan maintains: "Inactive people give aging a bad name." People think it's normal to look and perform 20-30 years older than necessary. "When they see a truly normal individual, they typicaly remark how young he or she looks," Sheehan observes.

Sheehan's (and Bortz's) prescription is this: "To restore life to your life, to defeat aging, to regain the youth you still possess, get your body in motion."

So I say, go for it. Junk your golf cart. Blast out of the zoo. Lace up your running shoes. Dust off your weights. Rejoin the hunt.

BORN TO BE LEAN

Why can't we follow in the footsteps of our ancestors?

Q: *With the help of your books and seminar tapes, I hope to reduce my bodyfat from 19.5% to 15%, and then to 12% (my long-term goal). Frankly, I was horrified to learn that my bodyfat is 19.5% (I had it measured by two different methods) because I lift weights and walk on an inclined treadmill four times per week. I am also careful about my diet.*

I'm 54 years old, and feel age is no excuse for having a high bodyfat. With some hard work and knowledge, I believe I can achieve my goals. Am I being realistic?

A: Relax! I have good news for you on all fronts. First, the average bodyfat for men your age is approximately 25% (30% for older women). Most doctors would not classify you as obese unless your bodyfat exceeded 30% (37% for women). Young men, however, average about 15% and young women about 20%.

Still, I agree with you that age should not be an excuse to gain fat. When I was 39, Lovelace Medical Center measured my bodyfat at 2.4% and almost 15 years later, when I was photographed for the cover of my new book *Lean For Life,* my bodyfat was again measured at 2.4%. So fat gain is not inevitable. With a little fine-tuning of your diet and training program, I am sure that you can achieve both your short- and long-term bodyfat goals.

Creeping obesity seems to be the norm in the Western world. The average 35-year-old male gains between one-half and two pounds of fat each year until about age 60.

Average need not be accepted as normal or healthy, however. Just because most people experience bodyfat increase with age does not mean that we should necessarily expect to get fatter as we grow older. According to *Exercise Physiology* (Lea & Febiger, 3rd Edition, 1991), the excellent text by William D. McArdle, Frank I. Katch and Victor L. Katch, there is probably no biologic reason for men and women to get fatter with advancing age. Many exercise physiologists now believe that there should be only one standard of excessive bodyfat for young and old alike (above 20% for men and above 30% for women).

One way to assess whether it is normal to gain fat with advancing age is to study the experience of our ancient ancestors. A team of doctors and anthropologists did that in a wonderful book called *The Paleolithic Prescription* (Harper & Row, 1988). The authors, S. Boyd Eaton, MD, Marjorie Shostak and Melvin Konner, MD, Ph.D., focused their attention on our genetic makeup, which was designed over millions of years and is largely unchanged in the last 10,000.

By far the vast majority of our ancestors survived by hunting wild animals and by gathering wild plants.

More specifically, the authors tell us that 100,000 generations of humans have lived as hunters and gatherers; 500 generations as farmers; 10 have lived in the industrial age; and only one generation has been exposed to the modern world of computers.

That's important, they explain, because the pace of biological evolution is glacially slow. Genetically our bodies are virtually the same as they were 40,000 years ago. In terms of genetic makeup, we are still hunters and gatherers.

Whether we are genetically programmed to get fatter with age, therefore, can be judged by looking to our hunter-gatherer ancestors and by studying the few remaining hunter-gatherer societies. The conclusion the authors reach is that we are born to be lean throughout life.

That's Progress?

The problem is that our natural tendency to be lean has been overcome by the drastic changes in nutrition and exercise patterns that have befallen our society in the last 100 years or so. Eaton and his colleagues observe that more change has occurred in the last 200 years than in the previous 10,000. In short, the foods we eat and the types of physical exercise we engage in changed, but our genes didn't. Our genes still "think" we are hunters and gatherers. Studying skeletal remains of humans from the Late Paleolithic period and analyzing the attributes of recent hunters and gatherers make it possible to develop a remarkably detailed anatomical picture of our preagricultural ancestors. They were very similar to present-day Americans in height. Their skeletal remains reflect strength and muscularity.

Significantly, the authors of *The Paleolithic Prescription* tell us that individuals in preagricultural societies do not gain fat and that they lose only a minimal amount of lean body mass as they age. Eaton and his colleagues conclude that the modern pattern of decreasing lean body mass and increasing fat with age is not natural. "It is the rule neither for people living in preagricultural societies nor among vigorously active Westerners," they state. Again, recent hunters and gatherers have been shown to maintain fairly steady body composition throughout life. According to Eaton and anthropologists Shostak and Konner, "This was probably the original norm."

What exactly was it about the diet and activity patterns of our ancient ancestors that kept them lean throughout life? How can our modern lifestyle be modified to keep us lean as well? To begin with, hunters and gatherers — both past and present — obtained all their food from wild game and uncultivated plants. Refined sugar — mainly honey — was available only seasonally. Roughage or dietary fiber was consumed in large quantities from wild, uncultivated plant foods. Although meat was prominent, the wild game they consumed contained about one-seventh as much fat as that found in domesticated meat. So their total fat intake was much lower than ours. As the researchers calculated, "To obtain 3,000 calories, hunters and gatherers had to eat five pounds of food, which kept their stomachs full."

More than anything else, that probably was the key to their leanness. The food they ate was physically bulky and dense in nutrients, but generally low in calories. Today, five pounds of some of our rich foods, the authors emphasize, can easily yield 9,000 calories. That seems to be the secret: to stay lean like our ancient ancestors, we should eat foods that fill us up without filling us out. That means we should emphasize whole-grain products, fresh fruits and vegetables, fish, poultry (without skin) and nonfat dairy products.

Exercise Or Die!

For our ancestors, exercise was mandatory. It was required for survival. *The Paleolithic Prescription* tells us that men commonly hunted for 2-4 nonconsecutive days a week, while women usually gathered about every 2-3 days. Like modern bodybuilders, they alternated days of intense physical output with days of comparative rest. The activities required for survival in ancient times promoted both aerobic endurance and muscular strength.

Translating this ancient fitness formula to modern times, the authors urge that we stay physically active through youth, adulthood and into late life. We should alternate days of resistance training with days of aerobic exercise. Finally, the authors suggest that variety — in both endurance and strength exercise — be the cornerstone of the modern-day training program. Such variation, they say, forestalls burnout, maintains enthusiasm and maximizes results.

Sound familiar? It should. That's the fitness formula recommended in my books and in *Muscle & Fitness* each month.

It boils down to this: to be truly normal — lean for life — adopt the lifestyle of our "caveman" ancestors. Follow the Paleolithic prescription.

CHAPTER TWELVE

THE LAST WORD

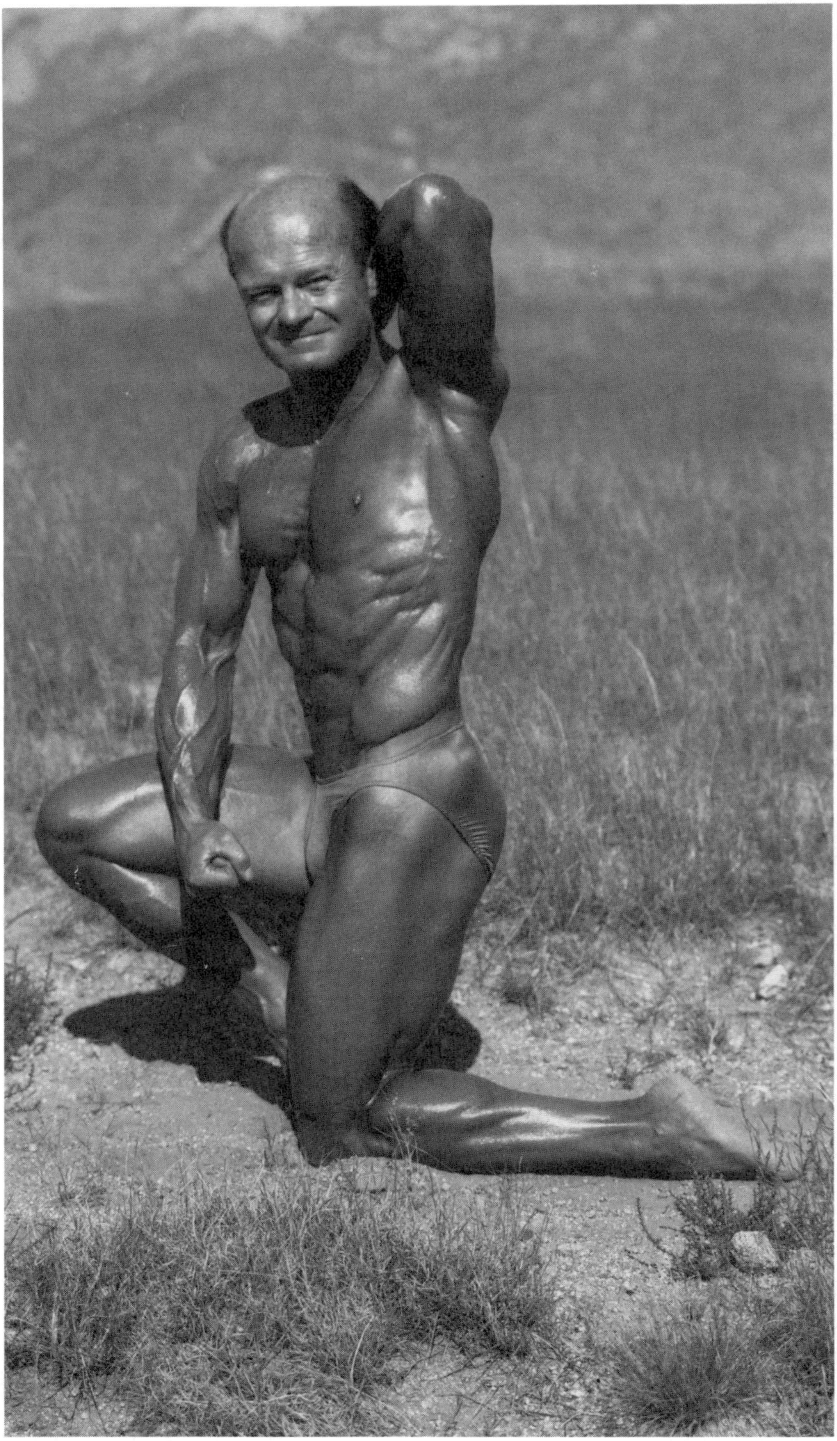

Photo by Guy Appelman.

THE LAST WORD 12

THE FOREST & THE TREES

Don't get bogged down in the details of sets and reps

My father always said, "The person who knows *how* works for the person who knows *why*." That saying came to mind recently as I talked to a good-natured but serious young man who had flown in for a weekend consultation. His local sponsor had told him that a contract with a well-known New York modeling agency would be in the bag if he could lose a few inches off his waist and add a few to his chest. It made sense, too, because he definitely had the clean-cut, all-American look.

A year earlier he'd lost 40 pounds. He burned himself out in the process, however, and, as so often happens, he gained back about half of the weight. He was determined not to let that happen again. Boy, was he ever determined!

"I have 200 questions for you." Those were the first words out of his mouth when I met him at the airport. I thought he was joking. He wasn't. The next morning when we sat down to talk he pulled out a legal pad with page after page of handwritten questions — 230 in all!

Fortunately, it took only a few of those questions to uncover his basic problem. He had read all of my books. In fact, he'd practically memorized them. He could recite what I had said in great detail. That was flattering, but it was also symptomatic of his difficulty. He was so immersed in the minute details that he often missed the main point. He didn't know how to extract the key principles of a program and apply them to his own situation.

He later told me that his mother also tended to focus on unimportant details. This recent consultation and some of the questions we receive through the mail and on the telephone lead me to believe that this is a common error. That being the case, I think it might be helpful to discuss a few of my friend's 230 questions.

Warm-Up

One question was about warm-up. Noting that in one routine I included two warm-up sets on the squat, he asked if he should always do two warm-up sets. In other words, he wanted a precise number of warm-up sets and reps for all exercises. I suggested that he stop looking for a fixed formula and focus instead on the reason for warm-up sets: to prepare your muscles and joints for the heavy sets, the sets that produce the results. "If you understand the reason," I told him, "you'll know that you should do as many warm-up sets as necessary, but no more." I warned him not to go overboard on warm-up, because that impairs your ability to do the sets that really count, the work sets.

End-Phase Push

In one of my books I illustrated an end-of-phase, heavy workout by having an imaginary lifter make a personal record in the squat by two reps. My friend wanted to know if he should always do two extra reps at the end of a phase. I told him that I thought he was missing the point, that the important thing is to overload the muscles in the final week of each phase. I explained that muscles grow bigger and stronger when new demands are placed on them. I told him that breaking new ground at the end of each phase will make his muscles keep growing cycle after cycle.

Then I asked him to consider again whether there was anything magical in doing precisely two extra reps. He shook his head and agreed that the key is to push to the maximum at the end of the phase. That, of course, might mean one extra rep, or three, or doing 5-10 pounds more than ever before. He was finally getting the idea that he should look beyond the reps to the reason for the reps.

Periodization

Let's look at one final question. My friend observed that in one of my books I laid out a periodization routine that divides the training year into three parts: a three-month high-rep phase, a six-month medium-rep phase and a three-month low-rep phase. This confused him because in a later book I described a different periodization routine. Have I changed, he asked. Which way is best?

I explained that *Ripped 3* contained my latest thinking on periodization. But I added that there are many different ways to structure a periodization routine. I told him that *Lean For Life,* my new book scheduled for publication in the summer or fall, contains further variations of the periodization model.

I suggested that more important than the specific details of any one periodization routine is the basic principle of following a routine until

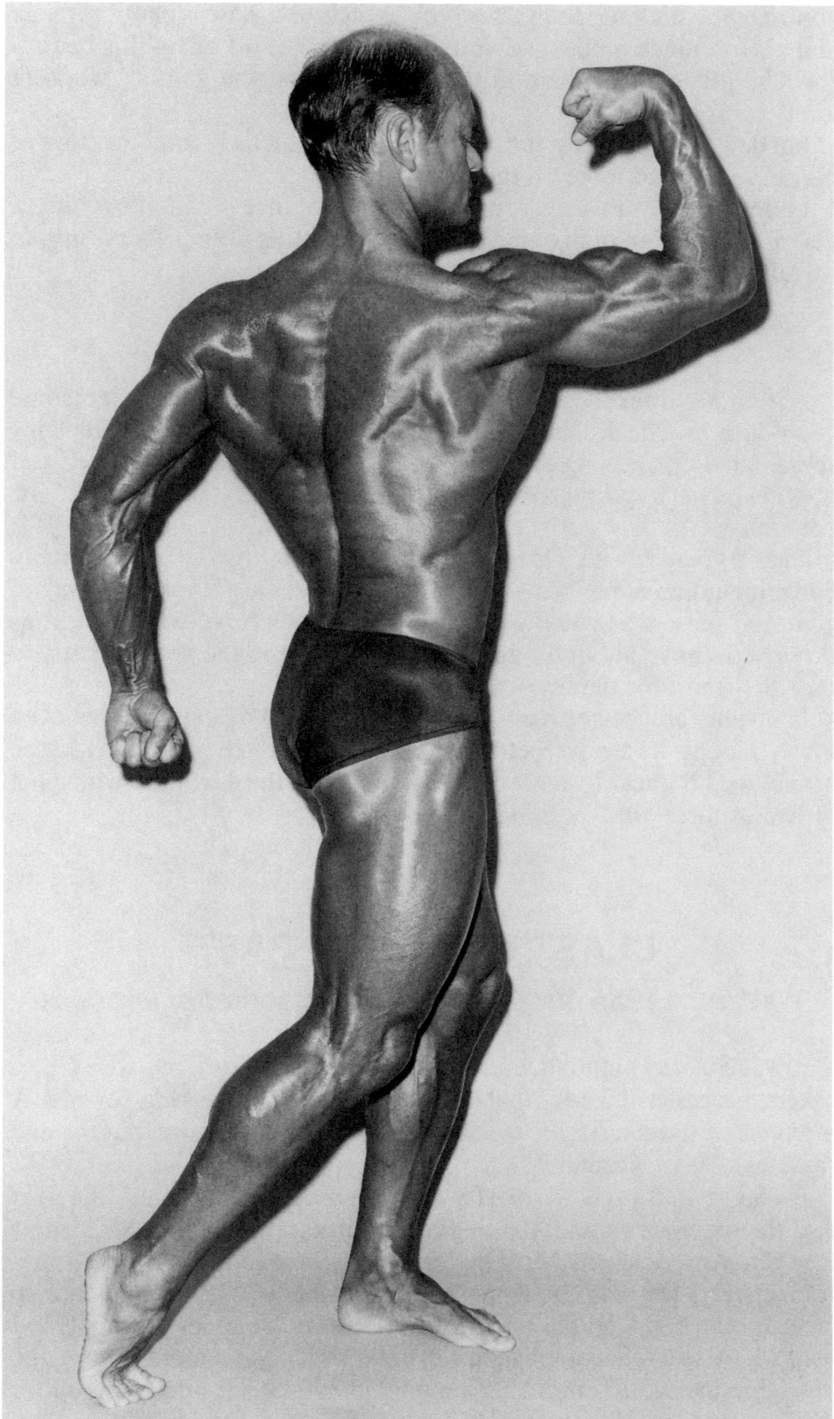

Photo by Dave Sauer.

you reach a sticking point; then you switch to a new repetition range and performance mode, and your progress takes off again! It's beautiful! The planned variation in this system keeps you gaining workout after workout.

I ended by suggesting that in the future he focus less on the how of periodization and more on the why.

I hope he takes this suggestion to heart, because it will allow him to get more out of anything he reads. He should stop taking everything so literally and try to understand the underlying idea.

No Blind Adherence

A famous track coach offered essentially the same advice some years ago in *The Runner* magazine. "I think it's a mistake to copy someone else's training program. Each athlete has different needs and abilities. The important thing is the principles of the program," he counseled.

That's great advice. One shouldn't blindly follow the advice in any book, including mine. Weigh and analyze what the author has to say. If common sense tells you it's good advice, adapt it to *your* special situation. And above all, don't get so bogged down in the details that you miss the forest for the trees.

I hope my advice helps my friend get his modeling contract, but even more, I hope he's now better prepared to analyze and solve future problems. I'll know I succeeded if he shows up the next time with a list of two or three vital questions.

BLAST FROM THE PAST

Visit from 1955 Mr. America recalls secret of success

It was Sunday night. "Can I help you in some way?" my wife Carol asked the caller. I knew that meant someone was asking for me. A moment of silence. Then, with a surprised look, she turned to me and said, "It's Steve Klisanin!"

As Steve and I talked, briefly on the phone and at length the next day, the memories came flooding back. Klisanin won the Jr. Mr. America, Mr. America and Mr. Universe titles in 1954, 1955 and 1956, respectively. He was the first "big-name" bodybuilder I met face to face. It was 1954, in the weight room of the Albuquerque YMCA; I was 16. Also an accomplished Olympic lifter — he rated among the top 10 in the world in the 198 pound class — Steve signed me up for my first weightlifting contest. I'll never forget it. Effortlessly, in slow motion and talking normally, he demonstrated the proper execution of

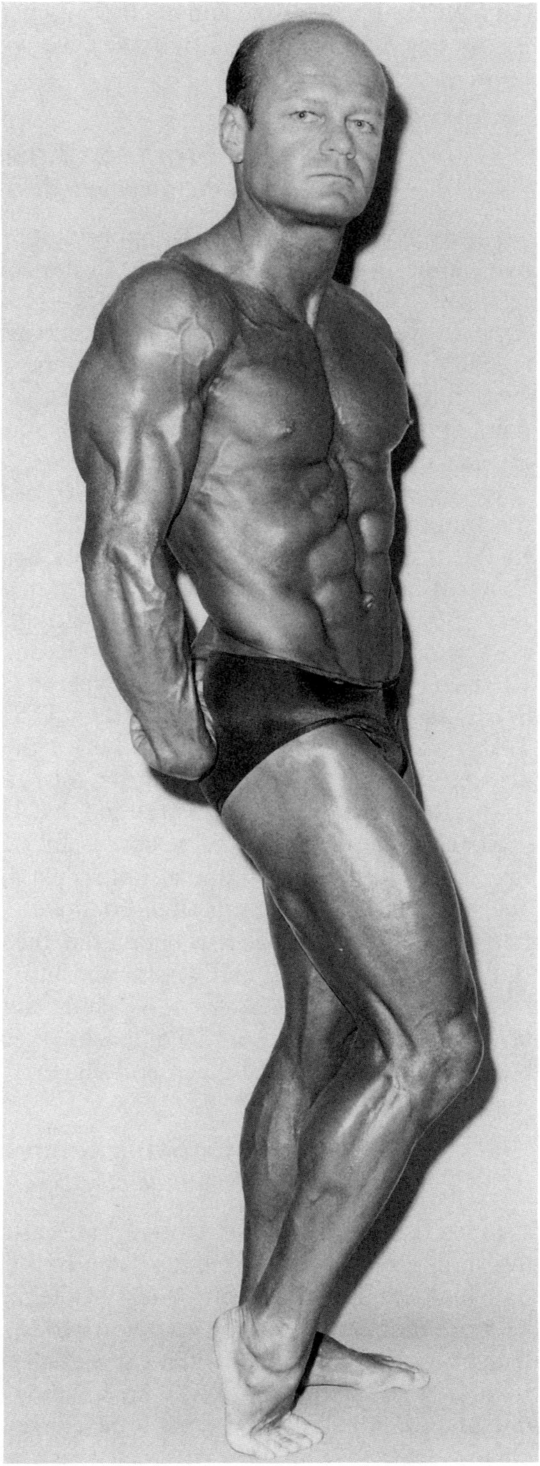

Photo by Dave Sauer.

the Military Press for me and my training partner — with more weight on the bar than we could lift. To say we were impressed would be a gross understatement.

Cue From Mr. America

Something I Needed To Hear

It was wonderful to have the opportunity to tell Steve the impact he had on me in my formative years. In the course of our morning-long reunion — it has been almost 40 years — I showed Steve a passage in *Ripped 2* recounting a remark he made to me, a biting remark. Understandably, he didn't remember the exchange, but I did because it was something I needed to hear. Tellingly, Steve's blunt comment made a point that two-time Mr. Olympia Dorian Yates, in his 1993 book *Blood & Guts,* credits as the secret of his success.

Here's what I wrote in a section of *Ripped 2* explaining what keeps me training: "About that time I went to an Olympic Lift contest in El Paso, Texas with the 1955 Mr. America, Steve Klisanin. At that contest I became one of the youngest lifters in the country to Clean & Jerk 300 pounds. That set my hopes soaring. I must have been popping off about the great things I was going to do, because I remember that Klisanin brought me abruptly back to earth. He said, 'You're no Norbert Schemansky.' (Schemansky was then U.S. and World Champion.) Taken aback, I asked Klisanin how he knew. I don't remember his answer but, as it turned out, he was right.

"I think Steve was trying to tell me that I should focus on state and regional championships and be successful there before I started thinking about higher level competition. That's what I eventually did. I became New Mexico champion, Southwest champion, Rocky Mountain champion and placed second in the Teenage National Championships and Junior National Championship. As a young lifter, if I'd refused to take the cue from Klisanin, and instead set my cap on becoming another Norbert Schemansky or else, I probably would have become discouraged and given up long ago."

Dorian's Secret

Do things step by step

In his post-victory tome, Dorian Yates attributes his success to having small goals and doing things step by step. He says a problem for bodybuilders is setting big goals while neglecting small goals in between. For example, they set out to add four inches to their arms and then become discouraged when gains don't come fast enough; they get frustrated and many quit. "It's like standing at the bottom of a mountain and thinking that you want to reach the top," Dorian explains. "If all you can see is the top, it gets a bit overwhelming because of the vast distance you must climb. If, on the other hand, you take one step, then another, then another, you're slowly but surely making your way to the top."

That's exactly what Yates did. His first competition was a novice contest, the 1985 West Coast Championships in Morecambe, England. "I walked on stage and the audience gasped!" At first he thought he had done something wrong, but soon realized that he was the clear winner. Importantly, Yates trained hard for two years before entering this competition. "I've always taken bodybuilding one step at a time," he says. In short, he prepared well for his first contest, which laid the groundwork and gave him confidence for the many victories that followed. He took bodybuilding one step at a time, obviously realizing the wisdom in the adage "Success breeds success."

Arnold

Aim high, but be realistic

It's fine, of course, to aim high. For example, soon after Arnold began bodybuilding, at age 14 in Graz, Austria, he turned to another bodybuilder in the gym and said, "Well, I give myself another five years and I will be Mr. Universe." (*Arnold* by Wendy Leigh, Congdon & Weed, 1990.) Arnold may be the exception that proves the rule, but still, like Dorian, he trained hard for several years before entering — and winning — his first contest, the 1965 junior Mr. Europe.

It's fine to know, in the back of your mind, that you'd like to be Mr. Olympia, or in my case another Norbert Schemansky, but you must remember that the longest journey begins with the first step. The strength of one's motivation depends, for the most part, on past success. To stay with it, bodybuilding or anything else, you must have success along the way. Again, success breeds success. Take a tip from Dorian and Arnold, as I did from Steve Klisanin, and plant your feet solidly on each stepping stone along the path to your ultimate goal. Do that and you'll not only rise as high as your potential allows, you'll enjoy the journey. Because as George Sheehan has written, "Happiness, we come to discover, is found in the pursuit of happiness."

So, Steve, thanks for the inspiration provided by your example — and for shoving me back on the path to success.

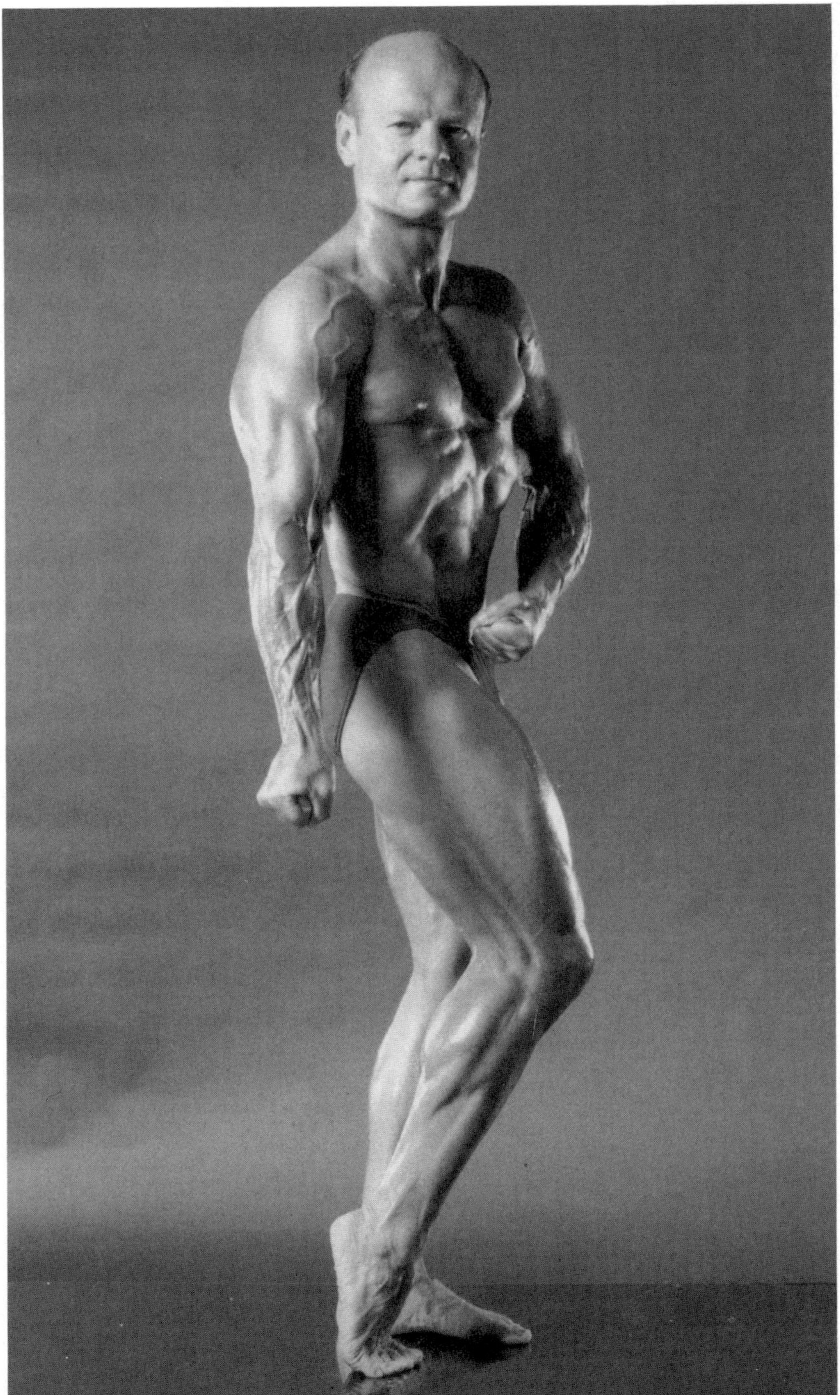

That's it, four more years. I'll see you down the road. Stay lean — and happy. *Photo by John Balik.*

HAVE YOU READ CLARENCE BASS' OTHER BOOKS?

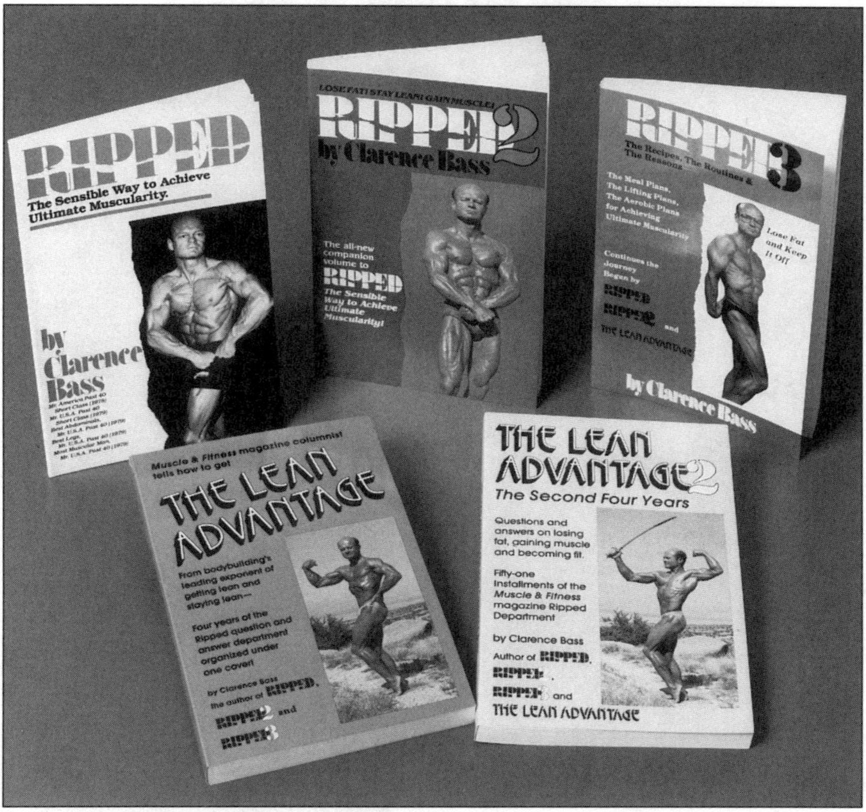

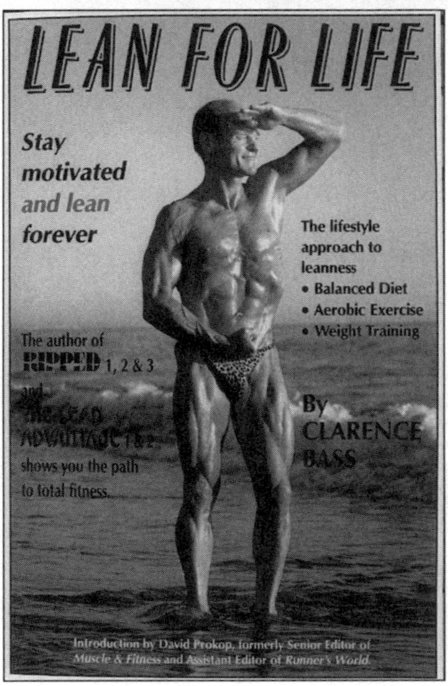

Please call or write for more information and prices.

Clarence Bass' Ripped Enterprises
528 Chama N.E.
Albuquerque, NM 87108
Phone: 1-505-266-5858
Fax: 1-505-266-9123